Cancer and the God of Love

Melvyn Thompson

Cancer and the God of Love

SCM PRESS LTD

334 00291 5

© SCM Press Ltd 1976

First published 1976
by SCM Press Ltd
56 Bloomsbury Street, London

Filmset in 'Monophoto' Baskerville 10 on 11½ pt by
Richard Clay (The Chaucer Press), Ltd, Bungay, Suffolk
and printed in Great Britain by
Fletcher & Son Ltd, Norwich

To the patients and staff of the
Royal Marsden Hospital

Contents

I

Discovering the Disease

The nature of cancer

The millions of cells that go to make up a human body are constantly growing, multiplying and degenerating. This is part of the normal process of life without which no complex being could survive. Each day some two per cent of the cells will be replaced; some change quickly (e.g. the bone marrow and the hair), others take longer, and a few create special problems because they cannot be replaced. Thus if the body suffers a wound, new flesh will grow to replace that which is lost, but if a nerve cell (which cannot be replaced) is damaged then the damage is permanent. If this process of cell replacement were removed, then the life span of our whole organism would be the same as that of its most fragile cell. *There is nothing strange about growth; it is at the very heart of life.*

This normal process of change and growth is held under the strictest control by the body. For example, when a wound is healing, cells grow only to provide identical replacements for those that are lost. If for some reason the control system breaks down, the replacement and growth of cells becomes disorganized and a tumour develops. Initially it is microscopically small, hidden undetected among ordinary tissues, but as it gets larger it may start to interfere with the body's normal functions.

Tumours are sometimes called *neoplasms* (literally newgrowths). Most of them are benign and very common, including such things as warts and moles. Almost everyone has them, and they do little physical harm unless they grow to a point where they exert pressure on a vital organ. Some neoplasms, however, are malignant, and it is these that are classified as cancers. One

I

basic difference between a benign tumour and a cancer is that the former will grow slowly and remain localized, whereas the latter will spread and infiltrate other tissues. It will infiltrate first those tissues that surround it, causing local spread. It may then be carried by the blood or the lymphatic system, part of the body's defence mechanism, to other parts, where the individual cancer cells will start dividing again to form secondary tumours, called *metastases*.

Why should this change in the growth of cells happen at all? This is the big question for research. We know that each cell has a genetic code which determines the nature of its growth. If for some reason the code changes, then the cell divides in an irregular way, and in the case of malignant neoplasms the cells may become quite different from those of the tissue of origin. It is natural to seek environmental factors to account for these changes, and there are substances known to cause cancer. These are called carcinogens. Of the many relationships between these substances and cancer the best known is that between cigarette smoke and cancer of the lung. Numerous things are thought to be related in some way to cancer, in the industrial environment, in the type of food eaten, and in exposure to radiation or even to strong sunshine. Research into this complex issue is continuing. Some environmental element is indicated by the fact that cancers common in one part of the world are rare in another. Yet at the moment most of the results are of a tentative nature, and the attempt to escape from all carcinogens would require an ordinary person to stop living altogether!

There are three things that need to be said at this stage, on facts about which people are often mistaken. The first is that with only a couple of very rare exceptions *cancer is not hereditary*. Members of a single family may seem to have a disposition to contract disease in a particular part of the body, although this is by no means certain, but where there are cases of similar cancers occurring in close relatives the most likely explanation is that cancer is a very common disease, and the laws of chance dictate that sometimes more than one member of a family may contract it. Often, indeed, one hears this idea supported by tales of cancer occurring among members of a family related only by marriage, or living in a particular locality. Since cancer cannot be passed on, there is no reason why a person who has been treated for cancer and who is able to have a family should not do so – their children are in no way at extra risk.

Secondly, *cancer is not infectious*. Since, as has been described above, tumours develop because of a loss of control over the normal process of cell growth, cancer is not a disease that can be contracted by being in contact with the sufferer. There is therefore no need at all for the person who has cancer to use separate crockery or take other such precautions. Everything can continue as normal. On the other hand, there are forms of treatment which lower a person's resistance to infection. Therefore it is sometimes advisable to keep such a person away from those who carry common infections, because he or she is likely to contract a succession of coughs and colds from them. Notice that it is the person with the cold who is infectious, *not* the person with cancer.

Finally, some may think that *trauma*, such as a physical blow to the body (and especially the breast) may start a tumour. Certainly evidence could be brought to support this, but there is no way in which the tumour may be related directly to the trauma. One probable explanation is that a blow to the body provided the opportunity for the affected part to be examined and the tumour to be discovered. It is also understandable that a person will seek some simple explanation for the trouble once the cancer has been found, and the injury then comes to mind. We know that division of cells takes time, and that the tumour was starting to grow in microscopic dimensions long before its discovery and the blow that was thought to cause it.

The varieties of cancer

Since they arise from a change in the growth patterns of cells, cancers are classified according to the tissue of the body in which they have their origin. The seriousness of the disease and the nature of the treatment will vary from one to another, and it would be more accurate to describe cancer as a family of diseases or a type of disease. The following are some of the more common cancers.[1]

Lung cancer accounts for about 30% of all cancers found in

men, followed by those of the digestive tract (20%), the skin (10%), the urinary tract and the prostate (7% each). By contrast, lung cancer in women is comparatively rare (5%), the most common one in them being that of the breast (25%). They too have 20% of their tumours originating in the digestive tract, and 10% on the skin, followed by those of the uterus (10%) and ovary (5%).

Other well known cancers include leukaemia, a tumour of the bone marrow which affects the white cells in the blood, and Hodgkin's disease, a tumour of the lymphatic system. These, along with very many others, go to make up the remaining 25% or so of cancers.

Cancer cannot be called an incurable disease. Without treatment it is progressive, but with it there may be a halt to the progression. Early detection is most important. The longer a tumour can develop and give out secondary growths, the more difficult it is to cure. If a figure is quoted for the cure of a particular cancer, it is an average result, and will depend upon many factors, of which early detection is one of the most important. Since cancer is progressive, the only way to see if a person is cured is to remove all detectable cancer from the body and then wait. If there is no recurrence, then all is well. It is convenient, therefore, to indicate cure in terms of those who are alive five years after the detection and treatment of the cancer. When looking at these and other figures it is worth bearing in mind that if a person is run over and killed by a car the day after being discharged from hospital there is no way of knowing whether or not the cure was effective. The figures that follow were given in 1973 and the treatment of the patients presumably started at least five years before that.[2] This therefore gives some idea of the results obtained from the treatment given *eight years ago*. One would expect to find that in some cases the cure rate for a person diagnosed today would be better.

The cancers that respond best to treatment include those of the skin and lip (75% of patients survive for five years, followed by the salivary glands (70%), the larynx (50%), the uterus and breast (45% each), the thyroid (40%), the mouth and the bladder (35% each). Others do less well, including lung cancer –the most common form in men.

4

Against these figures might be set the following, which give some idea of what can be done today to cure those whose cancers are detected at an early stage, before the spread of secondaries.

Patients with stage 1 of cancer of the breast (localized disease only) now have an 80% chance of five-year survival, compared with 45% overall. Those with Hodgkin's disease, which fifteen years ago would have been invariably fatal, now have an 80% chance of five-year survival if the disease detected in stage 1, where it is confined to a few groups of lymph nodes. Patients with cancer of the uterus, which like that of the breast has an overall cure rate of 45%, also have an 80% chance at stage 1.

If nothing more, these figures should give some indication of the variable nature of statistics given for cancer cure. In many instances a more serious cancer at an earlier stage is better controlled than a generally treatable one at an advanced stage. It would be fair to say that about *one in three of all cancers are curable*. We are dealing with a serious disease, but one about which there may be some room for optimism, and in the treatment of which there is steady progress.

Symptoms and relief

Most people do not understand all the medical details of their disease and its treatment, and only become confused by the complex language of medical textbook. What they do know, however, is that they are ill, and that their illness affects them personally. First of all they may be aware of pain or discomfort, or find that they do not have their usual resources of energy. These are the symptoms that lead them to seek medical advice. They are the most obvious effects that disease can have upon a person, and they are the particular concern of the medical and nursing teams. It is generally recognized that medicine has two functions to perform for the patient – it should seek to cure the illness, and it should give relief from the symptoms. Relief of this sort is given at every stage, alongside the curative treatment, and is in no way reserved for situations where cure is not possible. Doctors assume that if disease is creating problems for the

5

sufferer then it is important to remove them. On the simplest level, if someone is taken into a casualty department in great pain because of a broken leg, there is a basic need for something to remove that pain, although in itself it will not remove the basic problem or help to set the leg.

This form of relief from symptoms is obvious to anyone, however scant their contact with the medical world. What is sometimes less obvious is that illness can have other effects upon the sufferer as a person, and these have symptoms that need to be removed alongside medical cure. One such symptom is the shock of being removed from the familiar pattern of working life to enter the strange world of doctors and hospitals. With it can go the feeling that everything that gives life meaning has been removed. Another is the strain and bewilderment that can be generated with the family relationships when one member becomes ill. This is seen most starkly in the case of a sick child, and will be explored later in this book.

These and many other personal effects may be overlooked simply because medicine is dominated by the scientific outlook which concentrates, with good effect, on the physical symptoms, but assumes that what does not appear on an X-ray or blood test is therefore of little consequence. Yet sometimes these personal features of illness become almost more important than the disease itself, and the physical problems may be but a small part of the personal crisis that they have brought about.

If we attempt to relieve these symptoms we should guard against the danger of treating them as though they were physical. A pain is removed by giving the appropriate drug, but it would be unthinkable for a doctor to do so without also trying to find out what was causing the pain, if he did not already know. Yet this is exactly what is sometimes done in the case of personal symptoms! If drugs are given to sedate a person who is distressed there is little hope of finding out what is causing the distress – and the relief will last for only as long as the drug has effect. To remove a problem permanently it is usually necessary for the person to work through it to the point where he can grow to understand and overcome it. Each situation has creative and destructive possibilities within it, and in order to cope with a crisis it is important to understand these and

6

respond appropriately. Our task here is to set out some of the personal problems and feelings that may occur in the course of a diagnosis and treatment for cancer. The material has been gathered from conversations with many patients who have found it important to be able to talk about their situation.

The first signs of cancer

Many people assume that if a disease is serious then it will present itself in some dramatic way, and are therefore fooled by the painless and rather insignificant ways in which some tumours present themselves; and although some go to a doctor with a minor ailment fearing that it might be cancer, others show a surprising reluctance to accept medical help at an early stage. Some who get sick do not take any immediate action, hoping that the symptoms will vanish on their own. In part this may be due to fear, but it is encouraged by the contrast between what they actually feel and what they expect cancer to be like. In films and plays this disease appears in its terminal stages as often as not, and it is certainly better known through those who do not recover than through those who do. The assumption is made that if it is cancer then it ought to *feel* serious. At this stage the actual experience is *contrasted* with the imagined sufferings from cancer, and incredulity sets in.

The first step on the road to treatment is the local general practitioner. He is still regarded as omnicompetent by some, and patients go seeking the reassurance that all is well. Their illusion is shattered when his face shows signs of concern, and they hear him asking them to go to the local hospital for some tests. For a moment there may be a feeling that it is all happening to someone else. Then questions start coming into the mind – 'What does he suspect?' 'Why didn't he tell me anything?'

This feeling of uncertainty is reinforced at the outpatients department. Any questions will draw a blank. No one is able to say anything at this stage; it will all depend on the results of tests, and these will be sent back to the GP. It is quite astounding what can go through the mind of someone who sits around waiting for a routine test. Everything is unreal. Normally on a weekday morning he would be working, there would be a coffee break and a chance to chat. Now on this particular morning all his colleagues are talking about *him*: 'Poor chap, he's gone into hospital.' There is a sense of isolation, of having left the normal world. It is made worse by the waiting. During the working day there may be many demands on time, appointments to keep, people to see. Now, in this outpatients department, time doesn't matter. The staff assume that as a mere patient a person has all the time in the world. The only people who are publicly allowed to have time on their hands are the elderly, the chronic sick, children and the unemployed. A man may suddenly feel that he has been relegated to some secondary stream of existence, while the world moves on unnoticing.

Not only has his sense of time changed, but so also has the group with whom he is identified. In the department there is a single division between patients and staff, and it is natural to look round and wonder what is wrong with everyone else. He may have the rather comforting recognition that there are others who are worse than himself, or even feel a little superior that he can walk around unaided, but against this is the general sense of being a patient, as opposed to the busy professional person who walked through the hospital doors an hour or so before.

With time and a change of situation a person's mind can go to town on the possibilities that may spring from the tests. In a few moments all life can be seen as leading up to this particular situation. The results could show that there is a fatal disease, and he starts planning out how everyone will react to the news, what will be said, what the funeral arrangements will be. Some people try to escape from their thoughts and the whole situation by attempting to read a magazine, but more often than not it becomes something to hide behind, in order to give an impression of casualness. Others concentrate on little details in the room, vainly trying to deflect their thoughts from their own insecurity.

After the experience of being in an outpatients department for a morning, life can return to normal until the time arranged to see the GP for the results. Those few days can be difficult. At one moment the tests and experience of the hospital can seem unreal, some dream or figment of the imagination to be set aside and forgotten. In the next there can be a chilling thought that the results are soon to be known, and the whole process of speculating on them can start again. Throughout this period a man may have the feeling that what happens to other people, and especially to the more ill-looking of his fellows in the out-patients department, cannot possibly apply to himself. He may feel that illness must be kept away, reserved for those whose lives are less well organized and planned. As an extreme example of this, one elderly lady thought that disease was rather below her social standing. 'You don't understand,' she said to me. 'This situation is quite impossible! My father was a most influential man, this sort of thing does not happen in our family. I'm not like other people, and they just don't understand that in here.' Sometimes the recognition of one's own humanity, so obvious to everyone else, is very difficult.

In these first stages of the period before going into hospital we have isolated three types of feelings:

1. The unreality of illness when compared with the normal patterns of life and work.

2. The problem of trusting and believing medical staff. So far there is the GP and the staff of the outpatients department; more will come later.

3. The difficulty of accepting one's normality and humanity, and therefore recognizing that what happens to others can also happen to oneself.

These will be found throughout the whole experience of treatment, and the way in which the person has responded at this first stage may give a clue to understand how he will cope with subsequent stress.

When eventually the moment arrives to face the GP and hear the results, there is a double fear. The first part is that one will hear very bad news, and it is often countered by a desperate hope that all will be well. The second part is the fear that he will not say what is really the matter because it is too bad to be spoken about. The particular words in which this piece of information is conveyed make a lasting impression, and may often be recalled verbatim years later. The patient assumes that if the doctor knows something (which he *must*, since he has the results of the tests), then he must know everything. If he fails to answer a question directly, or says that more examinations will have to be done before a conclusion can be reached, then he is only playing for time and it would be better if he were honest. These thoughts may run through his mind, and with them come two questions:

How much does this person know?

Can I trust him to be honest with me?

This situation can become all the more difficult if ambiguous euphemisms are used. One person said of her doctor's description of her illness: 'Anyway, it's not cancer. It's something with a long name. He rather mumbled it, and I didn't quite catch what it was.' This may suffice for a first reaction, but later, doubts may return.

These problems will be magnified if a person suspects, or is told, that they have a malignant condition. Cancer is always better known through those who do not recover than through those who are cured; and this is understandable, since those who are cured, knowing the general misunderstanding about the disease, will fear being regarded as socially unacceptable if they admit to having had the disease. The patient may therefore have a one-sided view of the disease, and the GP cannot always help him, for the nature of the disease itself means that he will be able to say little at the initial stages about treatment or prognosis, but will refer to a specialist.

Waiting for hospital

There follows the final stage of waiting before admission to a general or specialist hospital. During this period there is a temptation to get all the information available on cancer. Since not knowing is the hardest thing to bear, people try to make their own diagnosis. *Unfortunately their information will almost certainly be out of date, and the possibilities of treatment which they see will be more limited than is in fact the case.* As we saw on the section on the nature of cancer, there are far more variables in a situation than the non-medical person can hope to understand, and the ways in which the treatment is used will vary from year to year.

Few books on the shelf of a general library are an accurate guide to the immediate possibilities of treatment or prognosis. For those who at this stage crave information there is the added problem that their endless talking about half-understood medical details may cause distress to relatives and friends, and may encourage the latter in the bad habit of always changing the subject – a habit which they may find difficult to break in situations later on where real communication about these things is essential.

Whether the reaction is to go through imaginary conversations with doctors about the prognosis (and this is almost always imagined to be bad) or to block out of the conscious mind all reference to the hospital appointment, there is an *all-pervading sense of unreality* and the feeling that one is different from other people, singled out by virtue of having to enter hospital.

During this period it is important for the person with the suspected cancer to recognize that he is quite normal, and that needing treatment for disease does not change his value as a person. The biggest single factor in promoting this is the conversation with the GP. If, by his directness and sensitivity, he can create the sense of trust in his patient, then he will allow him to behave in an adult way and remain in control of his situation.

The patient may discover also a sense of comradeship with others who have had cancer, and may be reassured by those who are able to speak *briefly* and *positively* about their experience. Yet there is even danger in this, for each case is in a sense unique, and close comparisons can be misleading. Considering the great variety to be found in tumours it means very little to say that two people have cancer; their actual situations may be very different.

2

Treatment in Hospital

When a person knows that he is soon going to enter hospital he tends to speculate about what it will be like, and builds up a fantasy based on his expectations. This may be very different from his actual experience when the time arrives, and he will then have to adjust his ideas. In the stages before admission we saw that the fantasy was building up, created out of the images of what the person expected the sufferings of a cancer patient to be. This contrasted with the normality of the routine of life, and often also with the lack of any dramatic symptoms, causing a sense of unreality and disbelief about what was happening. This unreality increases when the person actually opens the letter telling him the date and time when he should arrive at a hospital specializing in cancer treatment. When the day arrives there is a great reluctance to see fantasy become reality. Many feel that they want to turn and run.

It is absolutely essential therefore, if a person is to maintain his identity and some semblance of being in control of the situation, that he should be welcomed into the hospital *as the person he is*. This may sound a little strange, but its explanation is simple. In the fantasy about what it will all be like the patient may see himself or herself as a frail, sick person, helplessly lying in bed. His old self is left behind as something belonging to the world outside hospital, and this loss of self is like a little death. As the label is attached to his wrist giving his details and hospital number, and he sees his outdoor clothes being packed into a suitcase to be taken home, the new patient can feel that all normal life has come to a halt and that the future is uncertain and under the control of strangers.

One way for the hospital to counter this is to welcome new

patients as unique individuals who have come on the advice of their doctor to seek specialist help in coping with a particular problem. Part of this welcome might involve knowing the person's name and introducing him by name to at least one or two other patients and members of the nursing staff. This should happen quite naturally, as one would introduce a new person into one's home, without his being marched round the ward for formal introductions. The sort of questions that a person may ask on arrival show the desire for a personal approach. Information of the simplest kind about the ward and about one or two members of the staff whom the patient is soon to meet can be of great help in the first few difficult moments before he can be settled in a ward. It is important for him to know the name of the ward and how to find it; hospitals can be busy and bewildering places and can promote a sense of helplessness and loss. To know that there is a telephone on the ward can also be a great relief: at least the contact with the outside world is not completely broken.

Some people find it helpful in the first few minutes of their hospital experience to have some opportunity to explain, perhaps in considerable detail, some of the stages that have led up to their moment of arrival. It is a way of getting the situation into perspective. There is no need for comment to be made; all that is required is someone to sit and listen. This is facilitated also by meeting another person bound for the same ward that morning, so giving the new person someone with whom to identify, who understands what it feels like to have just arrived.

On arrival on the ward, fantasy and reality begin to come together. The person with reasonably accurate knowledge of modern hospitals, will find reality not too different from what he imagined and adjustment will be easy. On the other hand, if the ward is imagined in terms of some old war film with gory casualties being carried to and fro then the process of adjustment will take longer.

There may be a very good reason why a person behaves out of character when he or she arrives in hospital, and why feelings relate more to an impression of what the place might be than to the actual situation. Here is an example of such a situation, and it is by no means unusual.

A young married woman arrived for an operation. During the first three or four days of her stay, on the second of which she had her operation, she seemed to be depressed, withdrawn and emotional. She complained that the nursing staff and others were deserting her, and not giving her proper attention. 'What can I do? Nobody comes near, and I haven't seen a nurse for hours.' She could not be persuaded that the staff were in fact in evidence, although there was in fact a nurse in her part of the ward at the time. She insisted that she was being deserted and ignored. Gradually she started to take an interest in what was happening around her, and actually admitted that the staff were attending to her. She started to talk to other patients, and within a few days was walking round the ward welcoming new arrivals and trying to make herself helpful to the staff. She was able to reassure others that it wasn't at all bad to have an operation, and was keen to talk about her family and the small shop that she ran.

It was at this stage that the reason for her initial feelings of desertion became known. She had wanted to go to a local hospital but was advised to come to London. This advice had been welcomed by her husband and most of her family, who lived near to her in a little village community, no doubt because they wanted her to have the best attention available. For them, to go to London meant the hope of treatment not available locally. Yet for her it meant that they wanted to get rid of her, to remove her and the suspected cancer as far away as possible. At first she had accepted the advice, but on arrival had suddenly felt this desertion. The image of being sent away to die among strangers had dominated her first few days' experience, and her feelings about the way in which her family had treated her were redirected towards the hospital staff. As she began to realize that others were treating her normally, and that relatives and friends were coming from home now that the operation was over, she lost the image of desertion. Her usual welcoming and open personality came to the fore.

Because they are complex, there is no easy way of removing these personal difficulties associated with arrival in hospital. Yet in general terms, the more *personal* the welcome given to the new patient the more he is able to speak freely about his situation and adapt to it. There are many other features of hospital life that effect a person's evaluation of the total experience; here we can examine only a few of them.

Waiting

As in the pre-admission stages, there is always a time-lag between something being tested and the results being known, and it is during this period that the imagination has a chance to work overtime. The worst may be feared and the best hoped for. There is uncertainty about what is already known 'Did they get the tests muddled up? Did I get someone else's results?' This extends to the communication of results 'How much do they know *now*? Why are they ordering another test before they tell me the results of the last? Why are they hiding things from me? Are they simply confirming results too horrifying to speak to me about?' Living with this sort of tension and uncertainty is almost more unbearable than coping with the worst possible result. Very often a person will say, 'If only I knew, I could face it; it's this not knowing that is so unbearable.' Unfortunately it is true that with some medical staff this waiting for complete and honest explanation of results can go on into an indefinite future, and can cause untold personal suffering. With others on the staff there will be a desire to explain as much as possible to the patient in terms that he can understand. Naturally enough, this is the line of action which enables the majority of patients to feel most in touch with what is happening to them, and most able to rise to meet the challenge of the situation in a mature way. It also enables them to have more honest and open relationships with staff and with their relatives, for prolonged deception is a hard thing to bear and its discovery shatters confidence and trust.

Another aspect of the problem of waiting is sitting around. Even if the pressure of waiting for results is removed, much of a patient's life in hospital is spent waiting for an X-ray, or for a clinic to start, or for a visit from a consultant who is in fact on holiday! Always there is nothing to do but wait. This in itself goes against the way in which we usually value ourselves; for in

the normal run of life we are fully occupied and time is important, and the higher up the professional or social scale a person
is, the more his time is regarded as precious and to be allocated
with care. Now it is assumed that in the hospital ward the
patient has nothing to contribute with *his* time. All that matters
is *staff time*. Thus the business executive who by mid-afternoon
asks when he is in fact going to see the doctor whose visit was
expected in the morning, is told that the doctor is a very busy
person and will try to see him some time that day. He remem-
bers that this is exactly what his secretary would have said to
the junior nuisance who wanted to take up his time, and he
therefore feels himself to be in a situation where his concerns are
not valued highly.

*For a person who lives under the threat of serious illness, his time is the
most precious thing that he has. We all too easily assume that the
seriously ill person has all the time in the world; in fact he has less time
than others, and it is therefore more precious to him, and to be treated with
respect.*

Communication

Of the many problems of communication within hospital life,
the one that concerns us most in assessing the human response
to coming into hospital is the way in which information is com-
municated to a patient. A senior executive person can at one
moment be able to absorb quantities of information and make
instant decisions about it, and the next find that he is a patient
in hospital. Once there he may find himself being called 'Dad',
if he is senior enough to come within that age group, and to be
spoken to as though the simplest of things were beyond his
comprehension. Sadly, it is often up to the patient to assess the
best way to explain his IQ level to staff, and such explanation
may be seen by them as a threat. Many people who are termed
'difficult patients' have done little more than ask to be treated
in an adult way. Open and honest communication at an appropriate level is the means by which the individual person receiving treatment is given the message, 'You matter as an
individual, and I am here to be of service to you', rather than,
'You are sick, and may therefore be treated as a child.' This

may sound a ridiculous message for the patient to be hearing. What is more ridiculous, however, is that it is in fact the only message which explains the incredible lack of effective communication that is so often found. Such bad communication seems to be saying, 'While you are sick you do not matter as a whole person. Nevertheless, I will attempt to cure you so that you can again become normal.' It is a symbol which suggests that illness negates human value, and as such needs to be countered by every token of respect for individual persons. It is shocking that there can be within a profession that centres on human care and concern, relationships between doctor, patient and relatives that are based on deliberate deception. Fortunately there are many within the profession who see the need to change such situations.

Independence

Many patients, both men and women, find it difficult to come to terms with the fact that during their illness they are dependent upon others for all that they need. In itself the struggle for independence is natural and healthy, and it strengthens the determination to combat the disease and regain a normal pattern of life and work. Yet the sense of frustration, especially for those who have evaluated their lives chiefly in terms of their achievements on behalf of work or family, can lead to helpless resignation. One of the signs of this is the way in which adults can regress and behave in a childlike way in response to their restrictions, doing nothing without permission and taking no initiatives.

As an ideal of cure, the patient should indeed become independent in every sense. Yet no human being is really separable from those who surround him, and to evaluate life on the basis of contributions of a practical nature can be superficial. The period of dependence may therefore be of great service to some, by forcing them to acknowledge that they are accepted for what they are rather than for what they can do. Physical dependence is only a small part of the total give and take of relationships, and many a patient should recognize that he contributes much on a personal level to all who surround him, simply by being himself. To promote only a superficial independence does not help a person to recognize his basic need of other people.

Families

The strengths and weaknesses of various members of a family will usually decide who takes final decisions on matters of importance and who supports in times of trouble. It sometimes happens that the person who has held a dominant position in the family becomes ill, and for the first time someone else has to take charge. A powerful husband finds himself being organized by his timid little wife, or *vice versa*! This can sometimes be a liberating experience for the weaker partner, but it produces strain. Some patients feel that if they show weakness, then their husband or wife will be quite unable to cope; others are threatened by the newly discovered capacities of their partner.

Many of the family tensions and problems found in hospital are similar to those elsewhere. The disease and its treatment may simply have brought to a head a problem which had long remained beneath the surface of life in easier times. If the stress brings to light the problems in a relationship, then it also provides the situation in which some resolution of them can take place.

Fear

There will always be fear associated with sickness. It comes in three forms. There is fear of suffering and pain in itself, which is quite natural and can only be alleviated by the assurance that treatment will be given to counter these as they arise. There is fear of the unknown, which comes from the uncertainty of the whole situation. To a certain extent this also is unavoidable when dealing with serious disease, but it can be minimized by the promotion of trust between patient and staff through open and honest relationships. It is often thought that there will be fear of death within this category, but it is less prominent than might be imagined. Fear is often related more to the illness that might lead up to death than to the fact of death itself. Because death is ultimately certain for every human being, it is seen by some as a point of security marking the end of a period of total insecurity.

The third form of fear is that of failing to live up to one's own image. 'Am I going to look a fool? Am I going to break down and cry in front of him or her? Can I face the people from the office looking like this?' These are some of the questions that express fear of social failure, and they will be accentuated if the person has rated their social performance highly. All three forms of fear may be alleviated to a certain extent. The first by good medical and nursing care; the second by good communication and explanations of what is happening; the third by acceptance and respect for the person as an individual, quite apart from his or her social standing, and support to enable them to maintain healthy and open relationships.

We turn now to some of the particular problems encountered by the person receiving treatment for cancer in one of its three usual forms: surgery, radiotherapy and chemotherapy. Our concern here is not so much with the medical effectiveness of the treatment, which would require comment far outside the scope of this book, but with the total effect of treatment upon the person who receives it.

Surgery

This was the earliest form of treatment for cancer, and until the last fifty years it was the only one. This goes some way to explain the associations that the word 'inoperable' can have, for at one time an inoperable cancer was one for which there was no effective treatment. In almost every case, the first contact that a patient has with an operating theatre is for a *biopsy*. A small piece of tumour is removed and examined to determine whether or not it is malignant, and the result of this biopsy will decide what is to follow. For example, a lump in the breast is biopsied and, if found to be benign, is removed, leaving the breast intact. If it is malignant, the surgeon will need to proceed to remove part or all of the breast, extending his surgery to include all parts that might be involved.

Apart from the biopsy, surgery has two main functions. It may work for *cure*, removing the tumour and surrounding tissues. This may be all that is required where the tumour is small and there is no likelihood of spread. More usually it is followed by radiotherapy and/or chemotherapy in order to ensure that there are no tumour cells remaining in the body. A surgeon can remove only what he can see, or what he knows to be there through a diagnostic test, whereas the other two forms of treatment work on a cellular level, dealing with the tumour at a point where it may not be detectable. Surgery may also be *palliative*, which means that it can help the general situation without claiming to effect a cure. This may include the attempt to delay the progress of a tumour where it cannot be removed, or to give relief from pain or discomfort.

Alongside these two basic sorts of surgery, two specific functions can also be mentioned. Where cancer has affected a bone, that bone may break more easily, and orthopaedic surgery is required to repair such a 'pathological fracture', as it is called. Surgery may also be used to remove certain glands in order to change the hormonal balance of the body – which produces change for the better in some tumours.

Some hold the view that surgery has now gone as far as it is likely to go in cancer treatment, and that its future now lies in the perfection of techniques. Many new developments in treatment, although nearly always depending on surgery at some point, seem to indicate that the future lies elsewhere.

During an operation, the totally anaesthetized patient has absolutely no part to play in the work being done, and no control over those who are operating upon him. This constitutes our central problem. Before an operation the patient is anxious to know what is going to be done, and needs to have an explanation of what is involved and why it is necessary before signing a form of consent.[1] Where communication is good, and the patient agrees with the surgeon about the operation, in full knowledge of any alternatives that might be open to him, then as he lies on the operating table something is being done for him *with his permission and within the terms he has set out*. The surgeon is doing something that the patient would in a sense wish to do for himself but is unable to do. This places the unconscious patient as much in control of the situation as is humanly possible. There are additional difficulties where the extent of an operation cannot be decided until after it has started. The most common example, as mentioned above, is that of the lump in the breast. The patient generally signs a form saying that if the lump is malignant then the breast can be removed immediately. It implies that she will wake up after an operation without knowing what has been done, and many woman describe a moment of fear as they first look down at their bandages. Reassurance that the patient will be able to carry on a normal social life after a mastectomy, and that the operation will only be performed if absolutely necessary, may help to a certain extent.

Very few patients exercise their right to ask for a second opinion, or for an explanation of the alternatives to the proposed operation, or set a definite limit on what the surgeon can do; and it is generally because they are not sure of what rights they have, and feel overawed by the whole situation.

To those who fear that they will not come out of the anaesthetic, especially if it is their first operation, the threat of an operation is indeed the threat of death. There is no substitute here for a sense of trust between patient and anaesthetist, and reassurance can be given when the patient is examined and signs the consent form on the day before the operation. In general it is the sensitivity and level of communication between staff and patient that decides with what confidence and trust a person can face the operating theatre.

After the operation there is a period during which life starts to return to normal, marked along the way by little victories: the removal of drainage or stitches; getting out of bed; the first walk round the ward. The general feeling during this period can be most creative. It is a time when the body seems to be working to heal itself, and the efforts of the patient go alongside the work of the staff to give a sense of movement in the right direction.

In this form of treatment, parts of the body are exposed to radiation. This is done either externally, by getting the patient to lie under a machine which controls the source of radiation, allowing a certain amount to impinge on the body from outside; or internally, by putting a radioactive substance into the body by implant or applicator in a carefully determined amount and for a set period of time, thus radiating a specific internal area of tumour. In neither way does the patient become radioactive; he is simply exposed to a controlled amount of radiation, and is separated from other people while having it, for their own protection.

Although the idea of radiation causes fear, especially with the elderly, it is usually a painless form of treatment, and one which should cause no traumas once the person is familiar with the machines to be used. Ionizing radiation damages tissue cells, especially if they are in the process of dividing (*mitosis*), and some types of cell are more radio-sensitive than others. The aim of radiotherapy is to give doses of radiation to the tumour large enough to kill off the cancer cells, whilst doing minimum damage to the normal tissues surrounding it. This is often achieved by radiating a tumour from several different angles, so that the radiation is shared out among the normal tissues but concentrated on the tumour. It is usual also to give a succession of small doses, on the assumption that normal cells recuperate before those of the tumour, and will therefore continue to live and grow between treatments.

This is a most versatile form of treatment, and one that can be used at almost every stage of the disease. It may be used for cure, as indicated above, or in conjunction with surgery, either to reduce the bulk of a tumour before it is removed, or to ensure that no malignant cells remain in the surrounding tissues afterwards. It may also be used to good effect in the removal of pain or discomfort in some cases. Development of this form of treatment involves the use of more accurate and sophisticated machines, including the use of high-energy radiations (e.g. those produced by a linear accelerator) in order to deal with cancers that are too deep within the body mass to be reached by less powerful radiotherapy machines.

On the personal side, the treatment should cause no traumas once the fear of the large machines has been overcome, but it does create problems. A course of radiotherapy may be spread over a period of anything from four to six weeks, and will involve being under the machine for only a few moments each day. There is inevitably much waiting around to be done, and sometimes there are physical side effects, where sensitive skin suffers from 'sunburn' or where radiation fields effect the bowel action, causing diarrhoea. There is often a feeling of tiredness, and sometimes nausea.

The general feeling of tiredness and lifelessness that may build up during treatment, and continue for a while after it, is difficult to accept. With surgery the patient knows that something is being done and expects to feel the effects, but nothing is felt to happen under the radiotherapy machine and this makes the results the more difficult to appreciate. Feeling tired and having a lot of time on one's hands can promote a sense of depression and a belief that one will remain weak permanently. A young person who cannot raise the effort to do anything other than sit around all day may feel that he has become a case for a geriatric ward! Those who are told that these feelings are normal, and that they will pass in due time, may be able to come to terms with them more easily than those who assume that they are part of the disease and that they themselves are therefore getting worse. Reassurance and explanation of machines and their effects can be of the greatest significance.

Chemotherapy

Chemicals have been used in the treatment of disease for hundreds of years. All that is needed is to find a substance which can poison the virus causing sickness without adversely affecting the host body. An example from this century is penicillin, which kills bacteria by preventing the formation of their cell walls. This is possible because the cells of the bacteria are significantly different from those of normal body tissues. There are problems where disease is similar to healthy tissue – for that which kills the one is likely to kill the other – and this is exactly the problem with cancer chemotherapy. The cancer cells are not foreign to the body, but are a distortion of normal body cells. It is therefore important to find chemicals with a selective effect, leaving normal cells intact.

In practice, most chemotherapeutic agents have some adverse effects upon the body as a whole, and these effects are seen most clearly in the parts where the cells are dividing fastest (e.g. the roots of the hair and the bone marrow), and therefore involve the patient in having blood tests before treatment, and the possibility of losing his hair with some drugs. The side-effects of drugs are many and varied, and since a great variety of drugs are used in cancer treatment it is unwise to generalize here about the effects to be expected.

Chemotherapy has the advantage over radiotherapy and surgery that it deals with individual cells in almost all parts of the body. With both the other treatments there has to be some knowledge of the site of the tumour, whereas in theory it should be possible to treat a tumour of unknown site through chemotherapy. It is therefore particularly effective in containing disease which has already spread through metastases to other parts of the body. Generally speaking, drugs are given at set intervals of time so that they effect the tumour cells at a particular point in their reproductive cycle. In practice this means that a patient may come to the hospital once a week or once every three weeks to take a dose of the drug, staying in hospital if it is likely to cause nausea or other side effects. The drugs are administered by 'drip' into a vein, by injection, or by tablet, and the patterns for receiving them can be complex. On occasions a single drug is used, but more often nowadays there is a mixture of three or four agents working together. Chemotherapy may be used before surgery, to reduce the tumour to manageable size, or after it, to ensure the removal of all tumour cells. In this it may be used alongside radiotherapy. For some cancers chemotherapy is the treatment of choice (e.g. choriocarcinoma – a cancer of the placental tissues), but more usually it is used to control spread once the primary site has been treated.

Most of the personal problems associated with this treatment

24

are related to its side effects. It is reasonable to want to come into hospital if one is feeling ill and desperate for treatment; one comes in feeling bad and goes out feeling better. Unfortunately, the reverse is often true of chemotherapy! However effective it may be, what is actually experienced by the patient is a sense of being not at all bad at home for a couple of weeks, followed by a visit to hospital that might well involve nausea and general wretchedness. It is only natural, and to a certain extent valid, that the patient develops the feeling that he goes home to recover from the treatment he gets in the hospital. Expressions like, 'If I feel better when I'm not taking this stuff, then surely if I stop taking it altogether then all will be well,' or, 'How do I know that I'm not already cured and that they are going on with this beastly business simply for their own research?' are not infrequently heard. A credibility gap develops, not unlike that in the pre-hospital stage. Many describe the dread that comes over them two or three days before they are due to return for treatment. Since he is at home but frequently visiting the hospital, the chemotherapy patient is most acutely aware of the precariousness of his 'normal' life, and the disease is never far from the back of his mind. Many find help in talking about their fears and feelings with fellow patients, and need to be reassured and kept well informed about the progress of treatment.

Immunotherapy

We have looked at surgery, radiotherapy and chemotherapy as the three main lines of attack upon malignant disease. There are others, but they are far less common, and some (e.g. hyperthermia – where the body temperature is raised to the point where it is believed that tumour cells will be killed) have not proved to be of significant help in the curative process. One other form of treatment that is making headway, however, is immunotherapy. This is the attempt to stimulate the natural immune response of the body to attack and dispose of the tumour cells. This is especially worth exploring where chemotherapy may have killed off all but the last few malignant cells.

Since it is the failure of the natural regulative system that allows the tumour to start in the first place, it is reasonable to help the body to do what it should normally do for itself anyway. This has been used in conjunction with chemotherapy in adults with acute myeloid leukaemia with marked improvement over the results obtained with chemotherapy alone.

3

Three Difficult Relationships

Parents and Children

Cancer in children is rare. Figures from the Manchester registry of cancer suggest that on average a general practitioner will see *one childhood cancer in twenty years' practice.* Putting this another way, it could be said that each year, of *ten thousand* children between the ages of one and fifteen, *one* will develop a malignancy. Nevertheless, although rare, cancer is now the second most common cause of death in children in some developed countries (the most common being accidents). This is the result of the discovery of antibiotics and a large measure of control over those things that were the main causes of childhood mortality until recently. As with adults, we see concern about cancer coming to the fore simply because other illnesses no longer pose their threat to life. This is not the case, of course, in most underdeveloped countries.

In its many forms, cancer is still the same disease whether found in children or in adults, and the three usual forms of treatment are also used for the tumours of childhood. In their own way children may go through some of the problems experienced by the adult, and yet they adapt remarkably well to the routine of hospitals and treatment. The central problem concerns the relationship that exists between the child and its parents and the rest of the family. To this we will return in a moment.

The most common cancer in children, accounting for about 30% of the total, and the best known, is leukaemia, of which about 80% is the acute lymphoblastic type. Gliomas (tumours of the central nervous system) account for 17%; those of the connective tissue, including bone, about 12%; neuroblastoma (a tumour of the sympathetic nervous system) 8%; and Wilms' tumour of the kidney 5%. There are very many other forms of cancer found in children, including Burkitt's lymphoma, generally found in children from Uganda and reacting spectacularly to chemotherapy, and the rare retinoblastoma, a tumour of the eye which is known to be congenital. These go to make up the remaining 28%.

With these rare diseases each case is different, and it is unwise therefore to place too much emphasis on claims for a certain percentage cure. Nevertheless, here are three examples. In acute lymphoblastic leukaemia, 95% now go into remission with treatment, and the average survival time is about three years, with many surviving five years and a few now reaching ten years. In the less common myelocytic type the average survival time is still only about thirteen months. Of children suffering from neuroblastoma, 25% survive for one year and about 12% for five years. With the full treatment for Wilms' tumour – nephrectomy (surgical removal of the kidney), radiotherapy and chemotherapy – there is an overall claim of 60% survival.[1]

The particular problems of parents and children are therefore magnified by the fact that the disease is very serious, and even where there is a remission the parents may still go through the whole experience of loss and distress during the course of diagnosis and treatment. The problems of adults receiving treatment may also apply to children, but these problems are overlaid by the strong emotional reactions produced by the very idea of a seriously ill child. People sometimes protect themselves by being very hard and off-hand; one mother overheard a conversation in which she thought that she heard someone say 'that's the woman whose child's going to die', nodding in her direction, and it was at that moment that she felt most alone. Another described the way in which neighbours found it difficult to know what to say, and spoke of her child as though she were already dead.

The first and most natural reaction of parents when one of their children become seriously ill is to focus all their attention upon him or her to the partial exclusion of brothers and sisters.

After a while these other children may try to claim back a fair share of attention, often by being difficult, only adding to the general stress within the family. On the other hand, it is often the need to care for another child that enables parents to carry on and cope. Parents and friends may also feel the need to fulfil the child's every wish, with ridiculous spoiling and a change in attitude to money. Some children are given things appropriate to those who are much older, or are taken out of their usual routine of life on extra outings or holidays. On occasions the whole family setting is changed as the child's father takes time off from work to be at home. Most of these things are not done so much to benefit the child as to fulfil the deep needs of the parents, who feel helpless to change an unthinkably distressing situation. Along with this goes stress within the marriage relationship itself, with the intense frustration sometimes leading to violence or total breakdown in communication. Where the child does not live for very long the family will have a period of readjustment, both within the marriage and in the relationship that the parents have with their other children. Bereavement may be worked through for many years. On the other hand there is a danger that, even if the treatment is successful and the child lives, the results of emotional stress trauma, and loss of time from school may mean that the 'cured' child is intellectually and emotionally hindered in normal development. Helplessness and the inability to protect from a known danger are the central features of this difficult relationship between parents and their sick child.

In the hospital there are things that can be done to alleviate this stress partially. First of all parents should be allowed to speak freely about their fears and emotions (including their anger!), and if they wish to cry they should be able to do so in privacy and with the understanding support of a member of staff if this is sought. To be prevented from giving vent to feelings at such a time only increases the sense of helplessness and isolation. The key symbol here is *acceptance* – for the parent needs to be accepted and understood.

It is important also to give parents as active a part as possible in the running of the ward. They may want to cook special meals for their child, especially if they come from abroad. This enables the child to feel more at home, and also gives the parents some way to contribute to what is being done. Alongside this it is important to create an informal atmosphere, with nurses wearing ordinary clothes, and as many distractions as possible. The actual time spent in the ward should be kept to a minimum; and wherever possible the child should remain at home, receiving treatment as an outpatient.

The growing tension and loss of stability shows itself in many ways during the hospitalization. Family situations may change, and the maternal grandmother may suddenly adopt a predominant role, stepping in to take charge of the situation. She may do this in order to protect her daughter from strain, only to find that it increases her sense of helplessness. Feeding the child can become an obsession. If nothing else can be done, then rows of different drinks can be made to try and tempt the child to accept something, and the persistence in feeding can be carried on right to the end. Some feel that as long as the child can eat something then all will be well.

Guilt feelings are common. Parents can try to find some fault in themselves to explain why their child is suffering. This applies especially to unresolved feelings about the marriage, family planning, or the circumstances in which the child was conceived. *Acceptance and forgiveness*, with stress on the understanding of natural emotions at a time of loss, are the realities in which most find some comfort. They may never be articulated as such, but they will be evident in the way in which the ward life and medical interviews are conducted. If they think about it at all, most people visualize death for themselves in old age, surrounded by their children. This picture is turned upside down when the parent sees something of his own future being taken away in the death of his child. One father of a young man who was dying could not get out of his mind the single fact that he had been saving for years in order to leave something for his only son, and now he was being taken from him.

In this section we have looked at a particularly tragic relationship, and one in which it would be the height of folly to assume that problems could be removed by some counselling technique or rational argument. If such situations cease to create deep emotional stress, then we are no longer human.

Nevertheless we have mentioned several features of the experience, mainly concerned with the way in which parents are treated in the hospital, which can be used positively – as points in a mad and futile experience where something of true life can be found. Acceptance of themselves and their feelings; forgiveness where this is felt to be needed; a sense of being able to do something to help; these are some of the things which in fact enable parents to cope and somehow carry on living. They do not take away the pain from the relationship with the child, but they might help to make it bearable.

The dying and those who surround them

The heading of this section is misleading. *We are all at one and the same time dying and living.* To the severely depressed person everything is in decay; to the elated everything is filled with life, however short that life may be. This use of the two words 'living' and 'dying' may help us to decide between two attitudes.

If we choose to regard the seriously ill as 'dying', then we set them apart from other people as though they were different from the rest of us. We may adopt a different tone of voice in speaking to them, or even avoid all direct contact. They are not expected to take an interest in the usual pleasures of life, and if they seem bewildered or confused by their situation they are best sedated heavily so that direct contact with them is lessened. This all becomes a symbol of dying, of worthlessness and failure. It is a symbol of separation from life.

On the other hand, if we regard them as 'living', although recognizing that they may not do so for very long, then our approach to them will be different. They are like other people, with the same concerns and interests. Within their physical capabilities they will be expected to take an interest in life and join in things that are going on around them. What they are when living out the final part of their life is therefore only a natural extension of what they always have been. The aim of all who surround them will be to enhance such living as is possible. Where sedation is given, its aim will be to give relief from

31

distress whilst allowing maximum awareness and contact with people. It will *not* be a means of disposing with a communication problem!

If we were to speak out these attitudes, we would have to say something like this:

either, 'You are dying. You are not like me, for I am living.'

or, 'You are living; although your life, like mine, is fragile.'

Clearly, the second of these can promote love, acceptance, and wholeness of personal life (integrity), whereas the first is destructive of all these things. The symbol that predominates, whether it is life or death, will decide the nature of the experience for the sick person and those who surround him.

In looking at the fears that surrounded the diagnosis of cancer we saw that for many people it became a threat of death. They were faced with a situation of loss and meaninglessness, even if their condition was later cured. The same threat came over some who feared having a general anaesthetic for an operation. When a person comes to the final stage of his life he is not therefore facing a totally new experience. All situations of change and loss anticipate death to a certain extent – a death to what has given life stability in the past. How a person has reacted to these little deaths will give a clue to how he is likely to cope with the final stage of life and with the information about the seriousness of his condition.

Communication at this stage presents problems on all sides. The doctor may be reluctant to allow himself to be in a situation where the patient can question him at any depth, simply because it shatters his firm front of omnicompetence to face his medical 'failure'. Yet death is the natural end to life; why should he regard it as 'failure'? To do so sets the stamp of failure on all human activity, since we must all die eventually. It would seem more appropriate to speak of failure only in those situations where there has been a neglect of some aspect of personal care. One patient said to me, 'I'm sorry to let them down, they've done so much,' when she realized that she was not responding to treatment. Patients often seem to know more about the personal problems and limitations of their consultants in this respect than *vice versa*, and they make allowances for a lack of communication. It would be better to regard the final stages of life, along with respect and sensitivity over the matter of death and bereavement, as the *completion* of the work of the healing team, not as its failure.

When a patient knows the probable outcome of his illness (and everything is 'probable' rather than 'certain'), the questions that he wants to ask are often practical:

If I go home, can I come back into this ward if I need to?

You will give me drugs when I need them, won't you?

What will I look like? What will other people think?

Patients' main concerns include loss of human dignity, being isolated, being left in pain, and being kept half-alive by excessive medication. All such fears need to be countered by gentle reassurance, and the promise that as far as possible the person himself will be in charge of what is done for him. There is increasing awareness today of all these needs, and there is excellent written material available about it.[2] All that remains for us to do here is to put this situation against the general background of life and its personal values, to see how the one affects the other.

Those who say of illness, 'It can't happen to me,' often do so because they understand life mainly in terms of their external commitments and their plans for the future. Anything as human as being ill seems to have no place in their well-arranged scheme of things. The effect upon such a person of having illness thrust on him is often that it throws him back upon himself. He starts to ask, consciously or unconsciously, what he stands for as a human being now that he cannot hide behind his social or professional status. He may even start to feel that somehow much of what he has lived for has made his life hollow, devoid of human spontaneity. Now this situation is bearable if there is a chance of learning from it, and living differently in the future. There is a hope that things might change. But this is taken away in the case of serious illness in which the patient knows that there is little hope of recovery. *He is forced to face himself as he is, rather than as he might become.*

Every symbol and gesture which affirms the value of the individual needs to be used to counter the bewilderment that this causes. They will not be different from those that have given support and valuation earlier in life, making the person feel worthwhile; neither should they be, since this stage of life is only a continuation of what has gone before. Nevertheless the need for symbols of value in the *present* increases as the anticipated opportunities for change in the future decrease.

For those who are close to the seriously ill patient there is a mingling of physical and emotional problems. To spend long periods of time by someone's bedside, especially if he or she is unconscious, is exhausting. Time passes *so* slowly. There is a point where the relative or friend must get out for a breath of fresh air, or to have a meal. There may be children in the family who demand time, or other commitments to be met elsewhere. And yet the idea of being away from the bedside when something happens produces great anxiety. 'What happens if he dies while I'm out for a walk?' Generally speaking, the more the relatives can be involved with the routine of care the better. It is most difficult to remain in the ward yet feeling that there is nothing that one can do to contribute.

Not only is the person who is coming to the end of his life faced with accepting himself in the present, but the person sitting with him has to come to terms with their relationship. No marriage is perfect, and there will so often be guilty feelings in a couple about what they could have done together but did not. All the tensions in a relationship seem the more distressing now that there is less time to change them. In this setting, freedom of conversation with the patient, going over many of the things that they have shared in life, can produce a tremendous sense of forgiveness which on occasions may even need to be articulated directly. The final stages of life can be a unique time for reconciliation and personal growth for all concerned.

The cured patient and society

We have seen that some of the problems on a human level that occur during the diagnosis and cure of a malignant condition have physical causes, and these can be answered to a greater or lesser extent through medical and nursing care. Others concern the effect that the total experience has upon a person's way of understanding himself and his world. Most people have unresolved

34

problems which do not come to the surface as long as life moves on in its usual way unhindered by them. Yet a crisis or a personal threat can bring them out. It is therefore only to be expected that most of the problems encountered within a hospital will be those of society in general. For example, a person may be dissatisfied with his or her marriage relationship or general life-style, but will do nothing about it until faced with a period in hospital, during which the need to resolve such important areas of life becomes more pressing.

These problems are seen especially in the period of readjustment following discharge from hospital. Whatever the treatment has been, the patient will have had a profound experience, and one which sets question-marks against many of life's assumptions. On leaving hospital the patient has to relate this to the rest of life, and it may be some time before he returns to a normal level of social and emotional security.

The practical issue here is the quality of life that can be expected. Some patients will be able to resume their previous way of life, except for occasional visits to the outpatients department. Others will return regularly for chemotherapy. Practical help is given to those who have to face the fact of living with a colostomy, or women who need reassurance that they are able to look attractive and carry on normal social relationships after the loss of a breast. Many would benefit from the help of a counsellor of some sort during this period, so that their fears can be articulated in confidence and their questions about regaining social confidence explored.

Physically, many patients can set the whole hospital experience behind them, but there may remain the problem of how other people will treat them. All the fear and misunderstanding about cancer and its treatment, which in the first instance may have delayed many patients seeking medical attention, is now encountered again in terms of other people's suspicions. The cured cancer patient is still something of an embarrassment in society, and many pretend that their disease was something other than cancer. This only serves to complete the vicious circle, for the less they admit about their cure the less other people will understand and appreciate what is involved.

The key word here is 'normality'. The parents of a sick child find it difficult to treat him normally. The relatives of one who is coming to the end of his life find it difficult to treat him normally. Society in general finds it difficult to accept the cured patient as one who is normal. Unless the fact of disease and of the universal fragility of human life is accepted, it will always be difficult to resist the temptation to set apart those who live close to things which we most fear.

There remains another important post-hospital problem. If untreated, cancer is a progressive disease, and that progression is marked by the growth of secondary tumours (metastases) in other parts of the body as a result of the primary cancer. This means that cure or control has been effective at the point where there is no more malignancy. But the only test of this is time. With increasing certainty medical science is able to say that it has all been removed, but the proof of the pudding is in the eating, and the truth of the claim is only to be found in a normal life-span untroubled by recurrence. What is said to the patient is something like this:

As far as we are able to say, we believe that you are entirely cured. Nevertheless for your own good you should have a regular medical examination. As time goes on the intervals between examinations will get longer, and the chance of any recurrence of the disease will become more remote.

This is the eternal wait! It is rather like having a single premium bond; generally there is little chance of getting a prize, and if one does come up it is likely to be small and easily spent, but there is just the remote chance of the £50,000 win! For a long time no thought is given to the bond, then a list of winning numbers in a paper suddenly brings it to mind.

The same is true for the 'cured' cancer patient. There may be no recurrence. If anything does appear it will be noted at a regular check up and treated at an early stage, but there is the remote chance of a serious or fatal recurrence of disease in the distant future. Whenever there is an article in the paper about cancer, or a report about someone who has died from it, there is a sudden chill feeling 'That could be me'. Every symptom of a minor ailment now has a potential never before imagined. It is *not rational* to have one's life plagued by such fears, any more than it is wise to plan one's budget on the assumption that there will be a big win on the bonds, but for those who are by nature anxious it is a painful reality.

Such anxious people often find it helpful to be able to talk about their anxieties, and feel all the more desperate if they are prevented from talking about disease by other people who find such conversation difficult. Acceptance of the person along with their worries, and a promotion of trust in the medical team, may go some way to alleviate the tensions. Yet there are people who will always be anxious about something, and this must be accepted.

4

The Human Symbols

Many of the features of hospital life already described may be called 'symbolic', in that they point beyond the immediate situation in which the patient finds himself to the unseen values at the very roots of his existence. Everyone, whether or not he is religious, has some scale of values, conscious or unconscious, by which he understands and evaluates his experience of life. It is in situations of crisis, such as the diagnosis and treatment of a serious disease, that these values are put to the test and often profoundly shaken. Now if we are to help the patient who is going through such a crisis to cope with his situation, we shall need to enter imaginatively into the symbols that point to his values, to see how they can be used to support him.

No two people are the same, and their symbols of ultimate values will therefore also differ, but some features will be found more often than others. Personal fulfilment comes when, among other things, people feel that they matter, that they contribute something to life, and that their place in the order of things is accepted by others. In the situation of disease this is threatened by pain, which tends to make the sufferer opt out of social relationships or require heavy sedation, and also by the disease itself, which ultimately threatens life and therefore takes away all the usual sources of security.

Pain and disease are in themselves *impersonal*, but they threaten the person, who can be helped or hindered by all the other parts of the experience. For example, if the patient in hospital is made to feel that he is a 'number' or an 'interesting case' of some sort; if he is spoken of in impersonal terms by a group of doctors around his bed, as though he were some piece of machinery with no means of participating in the discussion; if he is introduced to visiting doctors as '. . . an interesting stage 3 carcinoma of the . . .', then he may feel all the more remote and withdrawn. On the other hand, if he is greeted by name, becomes known to some of the other patients and staff, and feels that his presence on the ward might actually have something to contribute to others, then *these things will work as personal symbols that give value, countering the symbols of impersonal uselessness.*

Symbols of personal value are promoted by such things as the layout of wards, the way in which new patients are welcomed, the human concern shown during the admission and registration procedures, the introduction of the new arrival to those who are in adjoining beds, and the way in which members of staff introduce themselves. The gestures and the attitudes of those around, especially visitors and close relatives, will go a long way to reassure patients in hospital that they are of value, and that they are still the same individuals now that they are ill. All of these things, and many more, constitute the symbols to be found in the present moment, and some of them will point to things of hope:

'I never knew I had so many friends, just look at these cards!'
'I like Dr X, he always has a little chat with me while he does his examination.'

All of these things can produce a sense of personal well-being even in the face of physical suffering.

But alongside these symbols in the present there will be those of the past and the future. With time on their hands, often for the first time in years, patients arriving in hospital will find that events in their personal history are turned over and over in their minds, especially those associated with sickness. Some of these remembered experiences will be sad, and some will be creative. They symbolize to a certain extent what that person has become in his journey through life, and those that are remembered as life-giving and fulfilling may be symbols that can point to faith – they constitute for the individual the experiences of his or her ultimate concern. The question which a person needs to be helped to ask, although not directly in this form, is:

'What, in your experience of life, has been most valuable, most real, and most true for you? What in all of life is most worthwhile?'

The answers to such a question will be many and varied, and they give the opportunity in a conversation to look in the past for a moment of insight that may be lost now behind the dominating concerns of the present. Perhaps what will emerge will be a time when there was a sudden burst of energy, with marriage or leaving home for a new job. It may be an experience – a holiday or a particular film. It may be a person – the relationship with husband or wife, or some deep friendship. Whatever it is, it will emerge from a general conversation, rather than as the answer to a specific question. For example, there are many elderly people who still talk about the First World War with an immediacy of feeling as though it only happened a couple of months ago. For them it must have been a time of desperate tragedy, or of sorting out the real qualities of colleagues. For most who went through it, the battles of that war became symbols of suffering and struggle and comradeship which can never be removed from a central place in their understanding of life.

These symbols of the past, as they are remembered in the present, play an important part in the interpretation of what is worthwhile. Yet this is also true of the symbols of the future. Most people, especially while young, have images about themselves in the future. It may be that a person looks forward to some professional success, or a time when life is well controlled with no more anxieties. Often the images get pushed further back until they become some hoped-for peace and quiet in a retirement cottage. They suggest the values by which the person is to live in the present, and they give the motivation for change where they conflict with what is actually happening. These images are important for a sense of value, but they are also the most vulnerable. When illness comes it threatens to remove the future, along with the possibility of ever fulfilling its images. The reality of disease may be a great shatterer of dreams and plans.

Where a person understands himself mainly in terms of what he hopes to become, illness will be a great personal threat. The threat may be countered in one of two ways. Either what has been pushed into the future must now become a present reality, so that success starts to be rated differently, or else the future hope must be retained as some incentive even if disease dictates

that it will never be fulfilled. For example, a ruthless professional man, who sees the present opportunity only as a means of
getting more power in the future, has an illness that will not
allow him to expend the same amount of energy on his work in
the future. It might be right to lead such a person to more of a
valuation of himself in the present, so that he is not plagued by
frustrated efforts to do the impossible. On the other hand, a
young person at school may have a prognosis so poor that it
becomes unrealistic to have academic ambitions. It may be
unlikely that he will survive a university course even if he is
accepted for it. Nevertheless there are times when continuing
with this is exactly what is needed in order to maintain the sense
of value, meaning and purpose.

From this we may see that while two people can have the
same symbols of success related to the future, the value of these
symbols for the present can be very different. The symbols for
each individual person must be assessed and related to his or her
life; there can be no generalization in the matter of how they
are used.

The nature of symbols[1]

What are these symbols about which we have been talking?
What is it that makes an experience symbolic? We start by
looking at some characteristics of symbols in general.

A symbol *points beyond itself*. Therefore when you look at a
symbol you are in some way looking through and beyond it to
some other reality to which it points. In this the symbol is like
any sign. A sign on the side of the road may indicate that there
is a dangerous bend ahead. The driver sees it and starts to apply
the brakes, just as if he had seen the bend itself. All that he
actually sees is a piece of metal with painted markings, but for
him it means something else. If we call the actual material thing
that does the pointing the *symbolic material*, then we can say that
the attitude a person has to the thing symbolized is different
from that which he would have to the symbolic material. Let us
take a work of art as an example. A scientific analysis of a
painting shows only canvas and paint. It is symbolic material,

41

and in itself shows us little. Yet to see that material as a picture is a totally different experience. We see at once that the artist uses it to speak about something of beauty or human emotion; it can express a whole awareness of life.

There may be a distinction between a sign and a symbol. The symbol has *power*. It makes real and present that to which it points. Thus an expensive car is a symbol of opulence; it not only points to that fact, but it goes to make it true. A kiss is not merely a pointer to some other reality called love, it is a symbol which has power to express it and make it real.

This last example leads to another characteristic, for love is in itself invisible. If you ask someone to describe love, what he will do is give a list of situations or emotions which point to it. In other words, he will list the many symbols that make love known. *The symbol makes perceptible that which cannot be known directly.* This need not always be the case, for sometimes the symbol points to something that *can* be known independently – the expensive car can be checked as a symbol of opulence against its owners bank balance. Yet in the particular field of religious and human symbols this characteristic is very important, as we shall see a little later.

A word of caution is needed at this point. We may be tempted to ask 'How can I prove that this symbol is pointing to something real?' Unfortunately there is no way of checking this. If the transcendent reality were known directly, then the symbol would be made redundant. We simply have to work from what we know. *If this particular thing seems to be pointing to a truth for us, then we have to explore that truth without asking for objective checks.* There is no guarantee that the loving kiss does not hide less welcome intentions!

Even at this stage, some value in the discussion of symbols for our concern with human suffering may become clear. If the ultimate truth and reality for human beings is not known directly and independently, but only through the symbols in life that reveal it, then *our knowledge of what we call 'God' will come through symbols.* Instead of having an already established idea of God which cannot be questioned but must somehow be squared with our experience of life, we have a more positive task: that of exploring the symbols of meaning and truth for ourselves, in order to give birth to our articulation of what we call God. This puts theological statements on an experiental level, and relates them directly to attitudes towards life.

Symbols, like living organisms, grow and die. They grow as they are accepted symbolically and mediate the truth of life; they die as they fail to point beyond themselves in a way that communicates power, and become mere matters of convention. A person may have a deep experience, and the occasion of that experience may become for him a symbol for what is ultimately true in life. Yet he cannot communicate it to other people unless they too start to see that the symbol is also true for them, that it finds an echo in the depths of their own experience. Too many religious expressions, which for one person are living symbols of the truth and depth of life, can become for others meaningless convention, unrelated to their experience. No amount of description can make that symbol live; it has to be understood at a deeper level. No amount of description of the nature of a kiss will make it anything more than an exhausting attempt at artificial resuscitation until the person sees what the point is, and why it is being done at all!

Many of these things would be true of symbols in general, but in the specific case of religious symbols two other points need to be made. First of all, the religious symbol points to something *which cannot be known directly*. To say that something is transcendent implies that it goes beyond the literal listing of bits and pieces of experience, in an attempt to express the value and sense of purpose in life as a whole. This cannot be done with scientific objectivity. It is only as individual things and experiences point to truths that underlie them that we can start to be aware of human dimensions in life as a whole.

The other point to be made about religious symbols is that they express *that which is implied in the religious act*. They come from a moment when there is a sudden intuition about the meaning and purpose of everything, and they are therefore reckoned as true or false depending on whether or not they can express that intuition.

All that we need to bear in mind for the purpose of our study is that the infinite, or ultimate, cannot be known in itself. It is experienced in and through situations which are called moments of religious experience. These moments have within them symbols – finite things, actions or situations in which the ultimate is revealed in and through the stuff of ordinary life.

There are different kinds of religious symbols, and they may be divided into two groups, primary and secondary. Of the primary symbols there are three levels. The first level is that of 'God' or the highest being; the second is that of divine qualities and actions; the third is that of incarnations – the holy seen in and through concrete things. Surrounding these primary symbols are others which resymbolize them so that they may be made real in different ways; they are secondary symbols.

The relationships here are illustrated in this example of symbolism:

> Devotion to the crucifix is really directed to the crucifixion on Golgotha, and devotion to the latter is really intended for the redemptive action of God, which is itself a symbolic expression for an experience of the unconditioned transcendent.[2]

Here the crucifix is a way of bringing something that happened in the past into the present. It gives an immediate awareness of the importance of that event when it is used in an act of worship. It is therefore a secondary symbol, whereas the crucifixion of Christ was in itself a third-level primary symbol – an expression of God in and through finite things. Yet that in itself expresses God's activity, and deepens an awareness of that which transcends and yet is at the heart of all life. Thus when we use one kind of religious symbol, there are many other layers to that experience which are also symbolic.

Let us now look at these symbols in a little more detail.

God – a first-level primary symbol. A religious experience contains within it an awareness of the *ultimate* truths and values in life. If it did not, then it would not be religious. Therefore one part of 'God', if we use that term to describe the object of our religious awareness, is the element of ultimacy. Yet it is also true that such experiences have a deeply *personal* character, and for many people there is a sense of being spoken to in a very personal way. This leads to a description of God in terms of a person. Literally this cannot be so, but *symbolically* it is a way of expressing the personal nature of ultimate truth.

In this way of seeing things, 'God' is not some being who might or might not exist. *'God' is simply the word or name that we give to the personal way in which man discovers the ultimate truths and realities of his life.* He is found, therefore, at the heart of the most personal human experiences, for those who want to speak in those terms. In no way is 'God' some theoretical truth about which there may be debate, and for the person who tries to stand back from his experience of life and look at it with scientific objectivity, all traces of the 'God' aspect vanish.

God's actions — second-level primary symbols. These spring out of the first level. They express above all the way in which awareness of the ultimate in life affects the individual. For example, the person may feel that there has been an action (God touched my lips and forgave me), or that there is a particular quality (God is forgiving), in order to articulate the liberating awareness of forgiveness at the heart of life. Notice that there is no objective test for the validity of these. They are true if they express the depths of the experience which they seek to articulate.

Religious objects — third-level primary symbols. Where something of the ultimate in life is perceived in and through some holy person, for example Christ or the Buddha, that person becomes a symbol pointing beyond himself. These third-level symbols are in fact the most immediate and common. They include almost all the examples of religious experience which we have given, and many will be found in the hospital. They are the things which point beyond themselves towards ultimate truth, and the previous two levels of symbols have largely been linguistic expressions of what is known through these third-level ones.

The secondary symbols. These are largely found within the practice of organized religion, and include all the ways in which religious truths are made present by religious object, gesture, or form of words.

Perhaps all the above could be summarized as follows. *There is a point where that which is transcendent and ultimate in life meets ordinary experience. That is the symbol, and from it springs religious awareness.*

In the religious symbol we have used a small part of experience as bearer of the meaning and dimensions of the whole.

Why can't all experience reveal these depths? In an ideal world everything would reveal to us its truth and its depths directly. There would be no need of religion, and no need to speak of 'God', for everything would be holy. Yet sadly this sort of experience is generally reserved for those called mystics, and most of us continue to value particular experiences and use particular religious words simply because much of life is superficial and does not reveal its truths.[3]

The symbol has its effect whether or not it is resymbolized in terms of God and his actions. Indeed, where the word 'God' is misunderstood, the attempt to use it may actually hinder the full appreciation of the symbol. For example, there may be an experience of love and of kindness which has the effect of transforming a person's attitude to life, releasing him from bitterness and resentment, and speaking to him of a quality of life for himself and others that he had long neglected. This could be resymbolized in terms of language about 'God' by saying 'God is love, and is the creative source of all things'. For some it might be useful to resymbolize it in this way, for others it might not. *Therefore the symbols are equally effective for religious and non-religious people, since there is no need for them to have a belief in anything prior to the effective action of the symbol.*

This takes the problem of suffering away from the restricted field of religious propositions and places it firmly at the centre of the experience of suffering for all. We use the process of resymbolization to link religious statements up with that which is actually experienced in life.

Symbols in hospital

Back in the hospital, the diagnosis of cancer in oneself or in a close friend or relative brings to mind many things. It becomes a focus of fears about the fragility of human existence. It symbolizes helplessness, suffering and death. It seems to negate all the positive symbols of hope for life. Now rationally many of these things may be quite inapplicable. The cancer may be cured or effectively controlled, it may be quite painless, and it may involve a minimum of time in hospital. Yet even if this is pointed out, as a symbol it seems negative in almost all its aspects.

The onset of cancer is therefore a point where a single powerful negative symbol seems to crowd out all other symbols of personal valuation. Interests, work-satisfaction, home and family all seem to recede into the background. If they were the basis of some faith in life, then that basis is now swamped by this new dose of reality. It is from this that the 'problem of evil' springs. Where human fragility seems to go against previously-held views of life, the person concerned may try to ask for a cosmic explanation. Why this suffering? What is its place in the order of things? A world which has to include this disease seems to make everything in life so futile.

The patient in the hospital ward is therefore in the middle of a conflict of symbols of self-understanding. Some good things earlier in life, which for a long time have given meaning to existence, are now in conflict with the present experience and symbols of suffering.

If there are to be found in our hospital situation symbols of healing and integration as well as those of suffering and loss, then we have a threefold task:

1. The negative symbols of fragility and death must find a place within a framework of life which also does justice to the positive symbols.

2. The implications of the present positive symbols must be reaffirmed and explored.

3. The question must be asked: Of these symbols, positive and negative, which do you understand as pointing to the ultimate truths about who you are as a person?

Once it is recognized that there are symbols in this situation, and that they effect people's attitudes, then we need to see how this can be used to help those who suffer.

It is important, both for secular counselling and for theological discussion, to start with those things which are in fact formative for the person's present state of mind. If a friend, relative or member of staff wants to help a person to change his way of looking at things, it is not enough to say that he is not being rational about his state of disease. Rational argument is not enough in these situations, since it does not answer the questions raised by the deepest feelings. Nor does it help to sedate a person who appears to respond irrationally to his situation – it simply ensures that the problem is never resolved. What is needed is a way of understanding the symbols that are involved, and the way in which the person responds to them, so that they may be *countered by other symbols*.

This point is vital. *A symbol cannot be removed rationally. It is no use to try to argue around symbols, for they are not created rationally, and they find their strength in deeper emotional levels of the personality. Rational arguments are too shallow. A symbol can only be answered by a symbol.*

A symbol of despair will only be alleviated by a corresponding symbol of hope. A symbol of fear requires to be met with one of trust. The task of the person who would be aware of symbols is to explore *all* the symbols that make up this particular person's attitude to life, and to allow some of the positive ones to take effect.

We shall see that the fact of disease, a particular tumour, is only a small part of the symbol of cancer. The power of that symbol is in the threat that it poses to life. Our task here is to help a person to maintain a positive and creative attitude towards life even through the most difficult situations.

The disease has provoked a crisis. It is being tackled on the medical level, and now it is right to attempt to help the crisis it has produced on the personal level.

5

Symbolic Therapy

A case study in symbols

We have already discussed in general terms the symbols that may be found in the hospital situation; however, because there is no such thing as the 'average patient', but only a collection of unique individuals in hospital, it is best to explore symbols as they apply to one particular person.

An elderly unmarried lady arrived in the hospital to be treated for a malignant condition. She appeared to be deeply depressed, spoke little and curled up in bed. When she complained of pain and general wretchedness she was given suitable medication but did not seem to feel any better. She couldn't care about anyone, least of all herself, and wanted only to lie curled up under the sheets.

Our first conversations were rather difficult. She said little, other than to complain, and cried silently. Gradually she started to explain her situation. She had been bereaved twice in the previous few months. Her mother had died, after being nursed by her for a long time, and soon afterwards her close friend, with whom she had lived for some thirty years, also died. Both had demanded all of her resources, and between them had monopolized her life to the exclusion of all other contacts. Her whole self-valuation had been in terms of those two people, upon whom she was totally dependent for emotional support.

Shortly after the bereavement, she found that something was wrong physically and sought treatment. Her condition was in itself quite serious, but was aggravated by her total lack of any incentive to live.

After a while she started to be drawn out of herself, and took

49

something of an interest in the other people in the ward. Their attention to her gave her the first signs of self-valuation outside the close trio of relationships so recently broken. Through them she started to discover a new environment within which she could live. This came partly through the close attention of the staff, and partly through the friendliness of her fellow patients. The situation on the ward became a substitute home, within which she had a part to play.

The difficulty came when the treatment was over and, after convalescence, she returned to her old flat. She was there on her own over the Christmas period, and experienced her bereavement most acutely. The new relationships with those on the ward could not sustain her, since they were limited to the time of her treatment, and she felt her loss to be quite overwhelming. She stayed in bed for much of the time.

During a later admission to hospital, she described to me the way in which it had suddenly struck her that hospital people come and go, and that she couldn't always be on the same ward. Therefore however much they had been for her a way of starting to live again during that previous autumn, she really needed something more permanent. She recognized that in choosing to ignore all other relationships in the past, she had created a situation which could not easily be changed, although she admitted support from some of her neighbours. She recognized that in a real sense her old life had come to an end with the deaths of the two people who had given it meaning. Although she did not realize fully the seriousness of her physical condition, she wanted to die, in order that she could feel at one with her mother and friend. She did not want to start another life. This was said with a sense of calmness rather than desperation, and it had been thought through deeply.

Her sufferings were therefore only in part related to the cancer, and it would have been totally wrong to assume that its cure would have solved all her problems. To the question 'How do you feel?' or 'What is troubling you?' she would answer in terms of the pointlessness of her life.

The problems and the suffering were to do with relationships that had been broken, and without which life seemed impossible. As it turned out, medical science did not succeed in

50

prolonging the impossible for more than a few months.

If the problems were of this kind, then we should expect the symbols of healing and integration also to be concerned with relationships. Let us now map out the symbols involved. The symbols of despair would include the sense of isolation, the recognition that she could not always return to the same ward, the temporary nature of hospital relationships, the memory of her avoidance of other relationships in the past. The symbols of healing which countered them included the relationships that were built up on the ward during her first admission (and therefore also the gestures and conversations that went to make them possible). These made her feel that she had value in herself quite apart from her previous relationships. Another powerful symbol was that of identification with those who had died. The part of her life that had given to them was something to be rejoiced in rather than mourned. She could feel that in a real sense she had completed her task in life. If there was no longer any future, then at least her life had not been a failure. She could look back and say positively, 'Yes, I did it for them.'

If we seek to know what belief in God might mean here, or where love might be found, we see that the cancer is almost irrelevant. It is the occasion within the normal processes of life that gave rise to the real suffering in terms of lost relationships. The issue of what was for her a symbol – a situation pointing to self-valuation and fulfilment – could be found by asking her 'What was it about those relationships (or that situation on the ward) that made you feel good again?' Her answers, in terms of gestures or the things people said to her, were symbols of *acceptance and love of herself as a person.* This already said something to her about life, in her situation of suffering; and, far from negating the religious depth, it pointed towards it. This is not to imply that in some way relationships in themselves are so important that they excuse lack of medical or nursing care. It is the giving of these that becomes a major symbol of personal care, but they need always to be combined with human sensitivity if they are to become symbols of personal value.

It may now be possible to give an outline of those things in the hospital which can become the basis of a positive attitude to life. First of all there is the context of healing itself. The fact that on the staff of a hospital there are people working together for the good of the patients may in itself contrast with some situations in life where others try to exploit or use people for their own satisfaction. The fact that there is a hospital at all becomes a symbol of care.

More specifically, the relationship of openness and trust that can be built up between a patient and a member of staff may be for *both* a real point of person growth. It symbolizes trust, acceptance and love, and makes them effective in giving a person courage to face physical problems. Friendships between patients on a ward may be profound, although of short duration, because of the very intense nature of ward life. These too may be symbols of acceptance, especially for a person who has previously had few real friendships. The way in which one is accepted into the community of the ward, and the attention received as friends arrive with flowers or gifts, have something to contribute to the total experience.

Symbolic therapy

One of the reasons for writing about the problem of suffering has always been to give the clergyman or counsellor some way of helping the sufferer to understand the personal implications of his situation, to come to terms with it, and to rise to overcome it.

Where this was related to belief in God, it seemed necessary to have some view of the world that could have a place for suffering and yet maintain an ultimate basis of love, making the person believe that in some way everything was going to work out for the best if only it could be seen in the right way.

Such a task was made difficult, if not impossible, in two situations. The first was that in which the sufferer had no real convictions about belief in God prior to the suffering, and the second was where the illness swamped all previous belief and the ability to think rationally. So, for example, it could have been thought that the function of theology was to provide a means of *arguing rationally* to a conclusion that would help the individual. A chaplain would be able to do his job as long as the patient was rational, and when this was no longer possible he could give sacraments to those who had faith, and trust in God's mercy for the rest.

Our situation now is totally different. It is not a new one, in that sensitive pastors have always been available for those with little faith, and have sought to comfort them in gesture, attitude and a willingness to listen to them on *their* terms. Yet this has been done with the rather general theological rationale that it follows the promptings of love and of service. *What is different now is the attempt to make this the basis of theology and not its by-product.*

'Symbolic therapy' is the term used in this study for the creative exploration of symbols of healing and integrity as they are found in the situation of one who suffers. It is theological in that it works with ultimate truths and values as they arise in situations that become symbolic, but it may be carried out by those of any religion or none, and *it is already being done intuitively by those who are sensitive to human dimensions.*

The basic principles of symbolic therapy, and the order in which they are to be explored might be set out as follows:

Stage 1. It is recognized that attitudes and religious comments may have their origin in some symbol, through which the person understands life and to which he has responded.

Stage 2. Where such a symbol works against what the person *wants* to believe, there is tension. This cannot be removed by rational argument. Indeed, argument of any sort may only make the tension worse, since it emphasizes the irrational power of the symbol and the feelings it generates.

Stage 3. The harmful symbol is countered by an equal and opposite symbol, which may be used to promote integration where it corresponds to the person's rational wishes.

The situation in the examples that follow is one in which the person is troubled about faith. There is a discrepancy between what the person wants to believe (or thinks he should believe) and what he actually feels. The attitude may have its origin in a symbol, which can only be found by allowing the person to speak about his tensions or about his faith, what created it and what may have shaken it. This will produce a story of situations which may be interpreted in theological language as symbols of

God's dealings with that person. As symbols emerge they are noted. The question to bear in mind is: 'Why has this particular thing become so important? As a symbol, to what reality is it pointing?'

As the picture of the person's attitude to life in terms of symbols starts to be built up, it is seen to fall short in certain directions. These may be the cause of the present tension. The symbols already present will need to be augmented by others, by bringing to the fore experiences from the past or hopes for the future which may then become symbols upon which his faith can grow.

Yet symbols are not created or destroyed rationally. *You cannot therefore create symbols. You can only explore situations and ideas in the hope that they may become symbolic.*

The hope is that in the course of a discussion something will suddenly become symbolic, and a balance will be restored. If the original problem was created by a symbol about relationships, then it is within that field that the answering one will be sought; if in terms of 'God language', then the answering symbol will also be about God.

Such an approach could be seen as a technique, but it should become what it has always been – the natural response of the sensitive listener, who prompts a person to explore certain areas of his experience. It is neither directive nor non-directive, but a mixture of both. It is directive in that the counsellor will attempt often to steer a conversation towards the exploration of certain areas in the hope that symbols may appear. It is non-directive in that it allows people to discover in their own way, and using their own terms, the implications of their experience of life.

The examples that follow are based on familiar comments made by those who are in a difficult situation, and they presuppose a general background of Christian belief.

'What have I done to deserve this?'

Here the suffering is interpreted as a symbol of punishment for something done wrong. It has two elements. The first is anger at the one who is doing the punishing, especially where it is felt to be totally undeserved. The second is a sense of guilt, turning over errors in the past that have not been forgiven, or for which punishment has not yet been administered.

The question may therefore be put in two ways. If the first element is predominant, it will have an air of defiance and self-justification: 'How dare I be treated like this? I've always been moral, and a regular attender at church!' If the second, then it will have a more depressed tone. 'Now I've been caught, and here comes the punishment. If only I hadn't done ... this would never have happened.' Where this is combined with a belief in God, his image is that of an angry father.

If this symbol of punishment predominates, then it will be used to interpret the whole experience of being ill. The problems of illness are compounded by those of isolation and victimization. Such a person believes that the real cause of the illness is far more sinister than the doctors imagine, and however optimistic they are, he remains depressed.

The process of therapy using symbols would start by allowing the person to speak about his faith (if it is presented in religious terms) and what created it. How strict was his upbringing? Was great emphasis placed on punishment for minor faults? Was there any situation in early life where he actually felt the reality of being forgiven for something? To what extent has his life within a church been a matter of appearing extra zealous or upright? Has he felt obliged to condemn others?

Naturally questions like these will not be asked directly, but they must be in the counsellor's mind as he listens to the story of the person's religious life.

Where the problem is not posed in religious terms, the process is still the same. The task is to build up a pattern of those formative ideas by which the person understands himself, noting in particular anything related to misdemeanour or punishment. Particular note should be taken where the illness relates to sexual parts of the body, for this is likely to enhance any idea of punishment. It may seem ridiculous, but elderly people may start to relate such illness to sexual activity half a century earlier! Guilt can linger at the back of a person's mind for decades, and an illness in the offending part is the natural punishment to expect.

55

Clearly, both in the secular setting and in the religious (which are the same reality described in two different forms of language), the symbol which counters guilt and punishment is that of *forgiveness*. If that symbol can grow, it will remove the sense of punishment and give a freedom, allowing the person to tackle the problems of disease in a more creative way.

We have already seen that symbols are not created rationally, and that it is not appropriate to counter them by argument. The person does not need to understand about forgiveness, he needs to *feel* it. The feeling of forgiveness may be promoted in two ways. First of all it may be possible to reflect on situations of forgiveness as they occur in the personal story, asking such things as: 'How did you feel when you knew that your friend had forgiven you for doing that to him?', or, 'Weren't you amazed that she still went ahead with the marriage after she knew about that?!' in response to what is said. The person may gradually remember what it is like to be forgiven, and recognize that it can happen again. It becomes a new part of life to be anticipated, and as gestures are made in that direction they find a response.

The second line of approach is to resymbolize forgiveness in terms of the present situation. As a person finds that he can say what he likes without meeting horrified condemnation, so he becomes aware that the person to whom he is talking accepts him unconditionally. Feelings which were not forgiven because they were never brought into the open and explored, can now be produced. As the counsellor *listens* and *accepts*, so forgiveness is actually taking place as a present reality. This is a common situation, and forms the basis of all forms of counselling.

This last idea emphasizes again the ordinariness of 'symbolic therapy'. It is nothing new, but it points to the symbolic nature of what is already known. This may then allow us to move from what actually works in terms of practical help to the symbols that underlie it, and thus to the theological issues that they express. In situations where the person seeking help is used to a more formal religious setting, confession and absolution are the normal run of theological therapy.

Some children learn that if they are good everything will turn out well for them. In adult life this may take the form of a determination to see the present difficulties out, confident of a happy final outcome. Yet this presents problems where the prognosis is poor, and the patient seems quite bewildered as things don't seem to be getting any better. How does this symbol of 'all coming right in the end' face up to the facts of illness and death?

As in the previous case, we start by building up our pattern of symbols by which the person understands himself, in order to see exactly how 'it will all come right in the end' fits into his general attitude. The symbols to look for are those which express triumph or beauty in the face of fragility. History and nature are full of examples, from the exquisite flower or butterfly that only lasts a short while, to the tragic hero of legends. The question in the counsellor's mind is: 'If you see this thing as beautiful although it soon vanished, or that person as successful in human terms although he died young, then why do you feel that life must always come right in the way that you want?'

For the religious person there is a wealth of material to be explored together. The image of the most complete and perfect human being suffering death on a cross is in itself a most powerful symbol of triumph in and through suffering, rather than of righteousness being an insurance against anything uncomfortable. How is this to be made real? Certainly not by arguing that if Jesus could suffer then so can anyone else. Rational argument is *not* part of the process. As these ideas and images are explored together in general conversation, the counsellor watches for the point at which a symbol starts to form, and the person says in effect, 'Yes, now I see it differently.'

A very simple example of this problem was given earlier in the book. The aristocratic lady who somehow felt that to contract disease was below her social standing, believed that everything had to come right for her. The symbols upon which she found herself reflecting, as she told me of her family situation, were exactly those of her most revered relatives who had suffered from all sorts of ailments! Without any argument, she gradually began to realize that illness was not a matter of social standing, and came round to seeing that her real problem was that of accepting help from other people and losing her treasured independence. This she had misdirected in terms of her own superiority. She came to accept herself more, as she identified with other sick people of her own background, including those that she had nursed in her youth.

'Why did God let him die?'

This, on the lips of a person recently bereaved, corresponds to the failure of the 'it will all come right in the end' attitude. Somehow the person who asks it is trying to find a place for death within a meaningful pattern of life. It does not seem appropriate to argue that God knows best, or that he has something better in store for him, for it is the failure of such rational thoughts that leads to the question being posed.

We need to start an exploration of those areas in life where human weakness and death are accepted as something normal, and not as the whim of some malign deity. The person may be encouraged to talk about other experiences of bereavement, or of encounters with death, in order that his previous feelings about it can be brought to the fore. Again, the question in the therapist's mind is: 'When have you experienced death as something normal, as an ordinary part of life?' Talking about the death of a pet can even provide symbols of naturalness and acceptance.

With this, as with many other situations, the basic symbol is that of *the one who accepts unconditionally*. Here the symbol has a double application. First of all there is the acceptance on the part of the counsellor of what the person wishes to say. Any anger or bitterness is accepted, and no attempt is made to change the subject. 'Why did God let him die?' may in fact mean, 'I feel angry and lonely, and I resent the fact that he has died, especially when I see other couples together.' Feelings like this can produce guilt and bewilderment. The acceptance of all this may allow the symbol of forgiveness to work. The second application of our symbol is the acceptance of the person who has died. 'Why did God let *him* die?' may have within it a fear that the death was a form of punishment. Some secret fault must have been discovered. In some way this may be related to the urgent need that the bereaved person may have of talking about the good qualities of the one who has died. That person needs to be accepted just as he was.

This acceptance of bitterness and questioning in the bereaved and of the person who has died, introduces a feeling that is exactly the opposite of that of being victimized, or found not to be worthy of a miracle. Bereavement is a very complex part of life, and to it there are no easy answers, but in general it might be true to say that support is found more in the symbols of acceptance than in rational arguments.

'All these things are sent to try us!'

On a literal level, this implies that a period of suffering can improve a person, and that God sends it in order to bring about something that would be impossible otherwise. This would be a reasonably positive way to understand it. It could also be taken as an angry expression of helplessness in the face of some force that is trying things out on us to see how we respond. On a deeper level, it may try to express failure to live up to an ideal, with the consequent feeling that this is to be rectified through an ordeal. It may express a determination to overcome everything and be strong, in order to prove one's own abilities. Or it may be a plea for help in a situation where one feels overwhelmed. This all assumes that it is said with a degree of seriousness, for it could be thrown out as a rather thoughtless comment in order to close a conversation. 'Oh well, all these things are sent to try us,' said with a shrug of the shoulders, can mean no more than 'I'm tired of talking about this subject, and the conversation is not getting us anywhere'.

On the assumption that in some sense it is said seriously, what are the symbols to be explored? They are those of positive growth and learning. The questions to be probed are: 'What have you learned through this experience? Do you feel that you are in some way strengthened personally through the illness? How have things changed for you?' There may well be symbols of growth that can be brought to the fore, and which give a new context within which the idea of illness having a strengthening effect can find a place. Where the comment has been an expression of helplessness, it might actually work to overcome it.

The above situations have centred on comments that may be made, using religious language, to indicate a personal point of crisis or tension. Recognizing that no two people are alike, and that the symbols of creativity and love will differ from one to another, we have attempted to indicate some of the areas which might produce symbolic situations. What will come out of those areas of life will then depend on the individual, and on the attentiveness of the counsellor.

For those who do not present a situation in religious terms, the same process can be used to bring their symbols of integration to the fore. In practice, the non-religious person often responds better to the prompting to explore symbols, since he is less tempted to look to the counsellor to provide a rational or 'religious' answer, and therefore more inclined to search within the realm of his own feelings.

The thoughts expressed in this chapter are offered on a tentative basis. They do not claim in themselves to do more than touch on some of the principles that guide all counselling. Their task within our study of the problems of suffering caused by disease is to provide a bridge between the counselling and caring (which in fact helps the patient to cope) and the theology (which explores what it all means in the ultimate human perspective).

6

The Traditional Problem
of Suffering

The question 'Why is there suffering?' has been asked in almost every culture, religion and philosophy. It seems to seek a rational answer. Yet we have already seen that rational answers, given by philosophy or doctrine, cannot in themselves penetrate the depths of the situation. Nevertheless it is important to look at a brief outline of the traditional problem, in order that we may see how our language about symbols relates to it.[1]

The problem starts with the idea that God is a being who is all powerful, able to do anything he chooses, to change any situation on earth, and to produce miracles where his will conflicts with the laws of nature. This God is then said to be a good and loving father, caring for his human children. His actions are therefore supposed to be for the good of those he loves. Against this may be set the fact that there is suffering and death, and that all sorts of horrific things caused by nature or man's folly continue in our world. The problem of evil in general may be set out quite simply.

> If God is perfectly good, he must want to abolish all evil; if he is unlimitedly powerful, he must be able to abolish all evil: but evil exists; therefore either God is not perfectly good or he is not unlimitedly powerful.[2]

For a person within the general Christian ethos of religious thought, love is such a central idea that a God who is indifferent is quite unthinkable. He is therefore likely to reach one of two general conclusions. Either God is allowing this particular suffering for some good reason best known to himself; or there is no God.

Where a person feels tempted to reject all ideas of God, there comes a further difficulty. What about all the good experiences and moments of insight that led him to his belief in the first place? Can they all have been an illusion? If God does not exist, then what does all the goodness and the love that stands alongside suffering and evil mean? The depth of such experiences of good will probably go a long way to decide whether the person rejects all ideas of God, or whether he simply remains agnostic about God's intentions in this particular difficult situation.

If this balancing of good and evil is a struggle for a person who has settled beliefs before encountering suffering, then the chances of one who has no such beliefs accepting them in the midst of such a dilemma become remote. If a person appears to have no faith when good comes his way, suffering will scarcely give it to him.

However rational or philosophical the question may appear, suffering is seldom thought about in a vacuum. A person asks 'Why?' in order to make sense of a situation. But he also asks it in order to find a way out. Language about God and suffering includes the idea of prayer and of miracle, and it is assumed that something can be done by God to change the situation, even if it is not understood why he did not intervene without being asked. A 'God' who is the result of an intellectual exercise may indeed give some answer to the problem of suffering, but unless there is practical help in the giving of courage and hope, such a God is no more use to the sufferer than the theologian who sits at a distance contemplating his plight. This has been expressed concisely by James Martin in his book *Suffering Man, Loving God*:

> The real problem of suffering is not the why but the how of it, not the finding of a satisfactory explanation but the finding of the means to meet it without being crushed.

and

> Even if a full explanation of suffering were available its real problem would persist.[3]

The great temptation for the person who suffers, when faced with a person giving a detached philosophical answer to the problem, is to say, 'Would you feel the same if our roles were changed? Would you still describe it like that if *you* were going through it? And if you did, would it help you?' A most moving study of pain and bereavement alongside theological debate is given by C. S. Lewis in *A Grief Observed*. His own grief brings to him a rejection of shallow arguments and a real testing of theology:

> Bridge players tell me that there must be some money on the game 'or else people won't take it seriously'. Apparently it's like that. Your bid – for God or no God, for a good God or a Cosmic Sadist, for eternal life or nonentity – will not be serious if nothing much is staked upon it. And you will never discover how serious it was until the stakes are raised horribly high; until you find that you are playing not for counters or for sixpences but for every penny you have in the world.[4]

However the arguments that follow are to be taken, and whatever the conclusions to which they draw us, the real test is within the situation of suffering itself.

What sort of answers can be given within the intellectual debate? At first glance there are two ways round our problem: either suffering has to be denied, or God is not all powerful.

At the one extreme it might be possible to say that evil does not exist in itself, but is simply the absence of a greater good (thus disease is simply the lack of health), or that all things are relative, so that what one person calls hardship, another accepts as luxury. Or we may have an idea of the world in which suffering and evil have a necessary and positive contribution to make. For example, a vision of evolution may demand that weaker species die off in order to allow the development of the stronger, or one of political development may allow violence and bloodshed as part of the necessary lead-up to a more peaceful and just society. Most of these ideas in some way allow the ends to justify the means.

Yet nothing is changed by saying that suffering is unreal. My situation as I lie in a hospital bed is not changed by some healthy person telling me that we are evolving to higher things, even if it is true.

If this is rejected, the other alternative is to suggest that at the heart of life there is a struggle between good and bad – two opposing gods. When evil comes, one side is winning, and when good returns, the other has exerted its influence. The forces of good are real but limited, and where they find suffering they struggle to overcome it, although they do not always succeed. This has much to commend it, especially in terms of practical action. Cancer is on one side and the medical profession is on the other; their struggle mirrors something at the heart of all life. Nevertheless, this denies the fundamental unity of life, and as such is rejected by many who want to retain the unity of God.

A position half-way between the two previous ones might suggest that there is a single good force driving the world forward, but that its progress is impeded by the natural limitations of the material through which it works. The force of life and growth pushes on the division of cells, and thus enables more and more complex beings to exist. Yet there is a limit at the moment to the regulation of this process, and where it goes beyond that limit a cancer develops. The cancer may be challenged and battled with, but it does not represent some independent malign force, only a sad distortion of the forces of life.

Reasons for suffering

The problem still remains that to accept an all-powerful God who is loving and kind means to believe that he *is* able to overcome all limitations and opposition, and that he therefore must *allow* suffering to continue for his own good reasons.

What might these be? First of all it is possible that suffering is a punishment, that it is inflicted on man much in the same way as a father corrects his child for some fault. If the child suddenly feels the smart of a slap, it is not his father's fault but his own, for doing the wrong that has deserved such a punishment. We saw earlier how this idea can dominate some people's experience of illness, and can hinder their co-operation with what is being done for them. To make sense of punishment at all, it must be assumed that it is better to have both sin and punishment than to have neither, for God could have removed man's free will and with it the possibility of failure.

If it is not a punishment, then suffering must in some way be allowed in order that it may be used for some better end. A person might be able to learn from it, or grow to overcome it. It provides an environment from which have come some of the most marvellous achievements in terms of human endeavour and compassion. All those hospital people would be out of a job if there were no more disease! How would we ever realize how wonderful health is if there is nothing to compare it with? 'Life is sweet when you think about the alternatives.'

If the first of these lines is taken, then the comments will be of the 'What have I done to deserve this?' variety. If the second, the 'All these things are sent to try us' will predominate, and a visitor might say: 'How do you know that through your suffering and courage others might not be learning a great deal, and that this is bringing about something wonderful that couldn't be done in any other way?'

Sometimes it is possible to see illness as a direct consequence of foolish action, as when a drunken driver injures himself. Sometimes it is possible to see good coming out of a tragic situation. William Marsden was motivated in his work by finding a young woman dying out in the street. Her suffering led to the founding of a free hospital service. Yet in the vast majority of cases, suffering is quite out of proportion to any recognizable benefit; and if it is punishment, then the one who administers it has some strange criteria of assessing who has done wrong, and even if it is deserved, his methods are those of a sadist.

Evil and the God of love

The conclusion reached by John Hick in *Evil and the God of Love* is that in the present there is need to struggle against evil as though it were an equal and opposite force, seeking to counter the good, but that ultimately the unity and purpose of all things will be revealed, and we shall then understand why all this is necessary.

If the definition of God with which the chapter started is retained, and if the reality of evil and suffering is not avoided, then some such conclusion is forced upon us. There must be some ultimate purpose in everything, but we cannot know it in this life. This may satisfy a person who has strong and settled Christian beliefs, for they will believe in some sort of future life in which they will meet God face to face and understand everything. Yet for the person who finds the idea of God a little difficult, that of the future life is hardly any easier. If he rejects the one then he will reject the other, and along with it the possibility of ever understanding his situation.

Seeing that there appears to be no rational answer to this problem, why is it struggled with time and time again? What is the real force behind it?

Let us map out here the sequence of events that might lead a person to have faith in a God, and later to ask the question about suffering.

A person may have an overwhelming experience of love and of acceptance. He may realize in such a moment that this is what life is for, that this is what makes the world go round. The ultimate nature of this intuition may lead him to say that he believes in a God of love. Following this, he may become attached to a church, or start to read theology or the Bible. Around his claim to believe in God will then grow a number of ideas which were not there in his original experience, but which he now accepts along with the belief in God. By way of example, his reading may lead him to say that God is all powerful and can perform miracles, yet there was nothing of this in his personal experience. *His* God was all powerful in the sense that he was seen as more important than anything else, and that he gave meaning and life to everything else, but this did not imply an ability to do miracles.

After a while the general acceptance of Christian belief goes far beyond anything that he had experienced. Most of it he accepts 'on faith', and sometimes he will be heard to defend it against the attack of sceptics. This he does because he wants to identify himself with the whole of the Christian group, and cannot base his belief on his personal experience only.

Later he faces a situation of suffering. The doctrines of God start to be questioned, and he starts to doubt if he believes in a God at all. Yet he wants to hold on to two things: the support of being within an identifiable group (in this case the Christian Church), and the original intuition about life.

He has two choices. Either he can struggle to defend the doctrines he has been taught, in which case he is in the midst of the problem of suffering; or he can reject those doctrines and explore only the implications of the original intuition.

The suffering may dismantle the set of beliefs that surrounded the original awareness of life. He can end up by saying: 'I don't understand anything about God any more. I don't know why he allows this. I don't even know if he is able to do anything about it. Yet what I do know is that love is still the most important thing for me, and even if everything else goes, that will be the thing that will enable me to cope with living.' He has lost the doctrines, but retained the fundamental truth.

Since it is our task, in the face of suffering, to enable a person to cope with it and to retain his own integrity, it is vital to find ways in which faith may be deepened and explored. *It is not part of our task to seek to defend doctrines; but only to work with the experience that those doctrines sought to articulate.*

These traditional arguments have been, for very many people, a source of great comfort, and if little weight is given to them in this study it is not to deny what they can achieve. Where they can help, well and good; where they cannot, we need to press on a little deeper into the symbolic heart of experience.

7

The Impact of Symbols

We saw in the chapter on the human symbols how an immediate situation could become a symbol, pointing beyond itself, and could be used to express convictions about life. These could then be resymbolized in terms of language about God, where this was felt to be appropriate. Thus the symbol provided a means of moving *from* situations in life *to* religious language, with the latter attempting to express the ultimate values for life as experienced in the former. In a hospital, some of the acts of care and kindness would become symbols of acceptance and growth, and would point towards love as a human truth. Yet other experiences would be impersonal and threatening, and these would become symbols of failure or worthlessness. Where we used language about God, it attempted to make clear what was already implied in the symbols. Yet it was an *optional* resymbolization, and where there was no talk of God the symbols still had their effect.

Let us apply this to the traditional problem of suffering as we have just outlined it. What has the idea of the symbol to contribute here? We saw that the literal definition of God as an all-powerful being, who behaved as a loving father, was seriously challenged by the facts of evil and suffering. Some who had held belief in God were tempted to remain agnostic. They could find no answer to the problem, and yet somehow wanted to retain the truth of that experience which had started them on the path of belief. Now with the symbol this becomes possible. If the idea of God is threatened, the symbol that produced it still remains valid. God-language is only one way of expressing the truth as it is experienced through the symbol, and where it becomes difficult because a proposed definition of God seems incompatible with the facts of suffering, then another way can be found. In a sense, this is exactly the position of the person who held on to his conviction about love and for the rest was agnostic. Any philosophical idea or doctrine of God can at most give only the *structure of thought* within which to articulate experience. It cannot give the *content* of our experiences and intuitions. Yet it is this content that is basic to any understanding and feeling about life. Except where illness has swamped everything, the question 'What is ultimately true for you? What is most of value?' can find some answer, even if all doctrines of God are found unacceptable.

Therefore our symbols can outlive the changes of philosophy and doctrine, because they do not depend upon them. They may use them, but they are equally effective without them. The rational arguments in the problem of suffering do not therefore render invalid the symbols of love and integration, nor do they hinder those symbols from pointing to the ultimate values and truths.

The language about God, as it comes through the religious symbol, is not a conclusion reached from the analysis of pieces of information. There is no need to add up all the good or evil things found in the world in order to balance the books one way or the other, and come to a conclusion about a God of love. It is much more to do with intuitions found in the heart of a particular experience, a matter of quality and depth rather than quantity. *The task of theology is therefore to articulate what is perceived in that moment of insight, and to relate it to the rest of life.* The actual experience or gesture becomes *symbolic material* pointing beyond itself to its ultimate truths.

This may be the way in which symbols speak of knowledge of ultimate things, but is it *in fact* true in most people's experience that knowledge comes in this way?

Two parables

To answer this, we turn to two parables given in the book *New Essays in Philosophical Theology*.[1]

The first concerns two explorers who find a clearing in which

69

they see flowers and weeds. They debate between themselves whether or not there is a gardener who comes to attend this clearing. Since they do not see a gardener, they devise certain tests, by which it will be known if he tries to come secretly to do his work. Yet these tests all prove negative. One of the explorers still insists that,

> . . . there is a gardener, invisible, intangible, insensitive to electric shocks, a gardener who has no scent and makes no sound, a gardener who comes secretly to look after the garden he loves.

To which the other replies,

> . . . what remains of your original assertion? Just how does what you call an invisible, intangible, eternally elusive gardener differ from an imaginary gardener or even from no gardener at all?[2]

The conclusion drawn from this is that the idea of there being a gardener dies the death of a thousand qualifications.

The interesting thing here is that the first explorer's conviction is held even in the face of mounting evidence of the fact that there is no gardener. He understands the mixture of flowers and weeds in such a way that he will hold on to his belief no matter how difficult it seems. This indicates that belief is much more a matter of looking at something in a particular way than of doing sums and reaching a conclusion from them. The two explorers have the same data with which to work, only their conclusions about it differ. The same might be true of two patients in hospital who have the same form of cancer, and the same domestic problems. Their understanding and interpretation of their situation may be quite different, as may be their ability to cope.

The second parable, this one by R. M. Hare, continues this way of thinking. The story runs as follows:

A certain lunatic is convinced that all dons want to murder him. His friends introduce him to the mildest and most respectable dons they can find, and after each of them has retired, they say, 'You see, he doesn't really want to murder you; he spoke to you in a most cordial manner; surely you are convinced now?' But the lunatic replies, 'Yes, but that was only his diabolical cunning; he's really plotting against

me all the time, like the rest of them; I know it, I tell you.'
However many dons are produced, the reaction is still the
same.[3]

Now Hare is suggesting that the lunatic has *a particular way of
seeing and interpreting things*, and this he calls a *blik*. The lunatic's
blik differs from that of normal people. In the same way,
religious belief could be seen as a particular *blik*; it could be seen
as a conviction about things which colours the interpretation of
all subsequent experience.

If this is so, then to a certain extent it renders invalid part of
the challenge of the traditional problem of suffering. If belief is
not a conclusion from all the data that a person receives, then
neither will it be destroyed if contrary data is produced – a *blik*
cannot be changed that easily. This may account for the fact
that there has always been suffering and evil in the world and
yet that people have continued to affirm belief in the ultimate
priority of love. The person who wants to believe will struggle
with all contrary evidence.

Yet if we accept that belief in a God of love gives a *blik* that
is neither created nor destroyed rationally, this is still only half
the story. Why is it that Hare's lunatic is afraid of dons? Why is it
that a person will affirm belief in God in the face of suffering? Why
should one of Flew's explorers continue to insist that there is a
gardener? If a *blik* such as this is not formed through an assessment of evidence, then at least *some* experience must have led to
its formation.

Here we have returned, by a different route, to the point at
which the symbol has its impact. *The symbol points beyond itself
and creates a new way of looking at life, which can then interpret all that
happens.* From the evidence of the two parables, something that
corresponds to the symbol would be needed for faith, even if we
had not started out to search for it. In some way faith must start
from a point of religious awareness.

The religious symbol

The religious symbol is a way of articulating that experience
which, arising out of the ordinary run of life, is able to give an

awareness of the transcendent dimension and values. It gives the starting point for faith, and from it there can develop a *blik*. Such religious symbols as we find within a hospital will give the strengthening points of faith. Yet this may be quite the reverse of what is to be expected. In the traditional problem, the fact of disease would be expected to go against any convictions and faith. Yet here there may well be points where the values of life are seen, even in the midst of physical suffering. For some these can be resymbolized in terms of 'God', for others there is no need to do so.

We have spoken at every stage of this study about symbols that point to integrity, wholeness of personality, and strength. We have assumed that love and acceptance are realities which are basic to a full human life. Naturally they have been related to the Christian faith, since they are qualities found in the life and teaching of Jesus of Nazareth. We have not suggested that the realities *must* work because they are Christian, but rather we have explored what does in fact work and then related this to the Christian understanding of life. Our study has started with experience and then moved on to the theology hidden within it.

Yet there is another problem here. By what criterion are we to say that love and acceptance are in fact basic to human life? How can we prove that isolation and hatred are less real in human terms? There is no way to do this, for rational argument cannot change a person's *blik*. Therefore if someone wants to take issue, and claims that disease and apathy are man's true goal, then this has to be accepted as *his* way of interpreting life. The only way of changing him will be through introducing him to that which is symbolic of love and acceptance for us, in the hope that it may also become symbolic for him – but this cannot be forced.

The ultimate question

In the hospital there are some things that point to despair and disintegration; there are others which point towards hope and care of the individual. Among all these conflicting symbols there is a battle going on between man and disease, both on the medical front through research and new treatment, and on the personal front as each person struggles to remain human. There is also a learning process, by which all who enter the hospital are challenged to grow to accept and overcome the undeniable fact of man's fragility. The question of faith, and of the symbols that go to make up a person's *blik*, is this: 'What is your ultimate concern? Where do you stand among the ambiguities of life? What do you hold to be worthwhile?'

Within a hospital there are *three possible answers*.

1. That *the ultimate truth lies in despair and disintegration*, and that all attempts to use positive and healing resources is against man's basic nature. This may be the situation of one in deep depression. There is no sense at all of identification with the struggles of doctors and nurses against diseases. Treatment is wrong and to be avoided, as going against human nature. Only in disease and death is the truth of man revealed.

I have stated this answer in its most stark form, in order that some of its implications may be shown. It is the logical outcome of promoting only the negative aspects of life, and making them ultimate.

2. At the opposite extreme it is possible to say that, although disease is real and not in any sense illusory, the truth about the relationship between human nature and disease is that *man is to struggle against it*. This is seen in the natural attempts of the human body to reject disease if it can, and also in the care and concern put into the work of medical, nursing and allied professions. Therefore the ultimate concern and the ultimate terms of reference will be the symbols of personal healing and well-being. These, rather than those of disease, are what is fundamentally true about human life. A patient with this answer will take his stand alongside doctors and nurses against the disease. (Yet this does not deny that there may be occasions where human valuation demands that treatment should not be pushed to the limits of medical possibility.)

3. The final possibility is a middle, non-committal path. Here *disease and healing are equally important or unimportant*. There is no identification with one side or the other in the struggle, and an indifference as to the outcome.

As a matter of fact, by observation, the vast majority of hospital staff and patients can be seen to identify themselves with the symbols of healing and integration. They see them as fundamental to their life; and, for those who are on the staff of a hospital, it was an identification with these symbols of healing which first led them into their career, and which sustains them in it. For patients it is the desire to be rid of disease, and to regain a normal pattern of living, that goes a long way to give them motivation to seek treatment, and to continue with it even when it is far from pleasant.

We might say, therefore, that for the majority of people a stand is to be taken firmly on the side of the symbols of love and of healing, and were this no longer to be the case then the hospital could not function. Neither patients, nor staff would have any inclination to join in the struggle. Where someone seems to seek only that which is negative, or seems indifferent to the outcome, he is assumed to be depressed.

Holding on to positive symbols, and working through them to help in a situation of suffering, is not simply to be equated with belief in God, but it is fundamentally the experience of such belief in a secular form. We saw in the section on symbols that God is a first-order symbol, and often therefore a resymbolization of some experience in the world that points to ultimate value and meaning. Language about God expresses that element of ultimacy, and what is said about ultimate priorities can be resymbolized and said about God. *Belief in God is one way of expressing ultimate convictions.*

If language about God expresses ultimate truths, then what we say about God reflects what we hold to be ultimately of value. Thus the statement 'God is good' requires for its basis the affirmation that what we know as goodness is for us, and therefore by extension for all, more true of life than that which opposes it. Acts and words of goodness around us are therefore symbols pointing to ultimate reality, and it is with them that we wish to identify ourselves.

The three ultimate options for the hospitals, as they were given above, correspond therefore to three statements about God. Where there is opposition to all that stands for goodness and healing, we can resymbolize as 'God is evil' or 'God promotes sickness'. Where there is identification with the symbols of love and caring, the statement is 'God is loving'. Where there is indifference to the outcome, the statement is 'God is indifferent'.

Notice, finally, that these statements are *not* propositions about what the world is like, to be accepted or disputed rationally. They are a resymbolization of those things which have become pointers for us, indicating truths about life. The affirmation or denial of such statements is a matter of life-attitude (or *blik*), and in this sense they are existential.

It would be true, therefore, that indifference to life and the statement that 'God is good' are incompatible on a personal level. Equally, a positive working for love and life is incompatible with the statement that 'God is indifferent' or even that 'There is no God', which is a resymbolization of the attitude 'Nothing is worthwhile'.

The 'How?' and the 'Why?'

There has been a division among those who are concerned about human suffering. Some have approached it from the 'Why?' standpoint and others from the 'How?'.

The 'Why?' people are motivated by philosophy or religion. They seek to stand back and survey the problem in an attempt to make sense of it. They look for some justification for all the problems and the pain. They feel that a situation can best be coped with once it is understood. It is the 'Why?' people who have struggled with the problem of suffering as it was outlined in Chapter 6.

Others do not pretend to be able to think through such things. They see that there is a situation of distress and they do all in their power to alleviate it. Their basic concern is 'How?'. How can pain be removed? How can this disease or that be cured? How can effective nursing care give a better quality of life for those who are seriously ill? Their motivation has been human compassion, and some have thought that the 'Why?' people could be better employed in useful action.

Between these two groups come the majority of people who ask both questions. Some have become so absorbed in the practical problems that they have been forced to ask why it should all be part of the world, if only to make sense of their commitment. Others have started with the philosophical questions and, without finding answers to them, have felt impelled to do something to alleviate the situation. Some may even have compartmentalized their concern, taking action in order to cover over a failure to reach an answer to the question 'Why?', or fleeing from the stress of direct involvement into the safer waters of philosophical speculation.

Certainly it could be said that, in general terms, a theological work is expected to deal with the 'Why?', and a medical or nursing work with the 'How?'. Yet this leaves both impoverished. If there is no ultimate perspective and reason for humanitarian concern, then there is danger of treatment for treatment's sake, and the loss of the centrality of the sick person in the excitement of medical research. Equally there is the danger that with the frustrations and difficulties of work, those with no ultimate perspectives may become disheartened. On the other hand, if theology and philosophy become separated from the real issues of healing and caring, then what good can they do for the sick person? Can a slick philosophical answer in any way change his situation?

In this study, through the theory of the religious symbol, we have attempted to bring together the 'Why?' and the 'How?'. The religious symbol is the starting point for exploring the depths beneath the surface of life. Yet the symbol is also the moment where an actual situation is encountered and help given. The symbols in hospital are the expressions of physical and personal healing.

Whether they are aware of it or not, those who are mediating symbols of healing and integration are producing in their work and attitudes the raw material for the answer to the question of man and his fragility. They are revealing depths in a situation which works to overcome the problems of man's finitude, and these depths are vital for self-understanding. Those who ask questions about 'Why?' will find their answers by involving themselves in the symbols that point to healing. We could sum up this chapter by saying:

'How?' without 'Why?' is superficial and lacks direction.

'Why?' without 'How?' is remote from life, and an intense frustration.

In the symbol, the 'How?' and the 'Why?' come together.

8

Some Conclusions

Our task in this book has been to explore what faith can mean for a person suffering from cancer, and how it can help him with his problems. In order to do this we have tried to look at the significance of disease and treatment for our understanding of life, both for the religious person and the non-religious, and have probed some of the human dimensions of hospital life.

In looking at the traditional problem of suffering we saw that the answers given were rational, attempting in some way to explain suffering, or based on a doctrine of the future life in which all would be made clear. Yet rational answers seemed too shallow in a situation of suffering, and acceptance of doctrines became difficult in an emotional situation which caused everything to be questioned. The answers given might support an already existing faith, but they could not be expected to create one, and all attempts to get an objective assessment of the place of suffering in the world only ended in ambiguity.

This impasse could lead to religious despair, with the question 'Why should this be so? Why *me*?' heard in emotional outburst, in silent determination, or in numb agnosticism towards everything in life. We therefore sought a theology of suffering that could arise out of the actual situation of disease and treatment, and could interpret those things which actually give hope and encouragement to patients. This we found in the idea of the religious symbol.

The symbol arises when a part of our normal experience of life points towards transcendent truths which cannot be perceived directly, and which can be resymbolized in terms of 'God'. *God is not a hypothesis, to be accepted or rejected with changes of data, but is the ultimate depth and truth about life as perceived in a moment of insight.* We found, in examining this, that the original symbolic experience could be resymbolized into language about God and his actions, for those who were happy to use such language, or made present through symbolic gestures and actions which could bring to the fore the liberating effects of the original symbol.

If we have a faith based on symbols, and if they can be used to restore it, as well as create it in the first instance, there remains one essential question to be tackled.

Are there symbols of hope that can create faith even in the physical suffering caused by cancer?

We looked at the actual situation of a cancer patient from the moment of diagnosis, and attempted to enter imaginatively into the feelings that were involved, and the experiences through which he would pass in the course of receiving treatment. We found that there could be within a hospital elements of trust, hope, acceptance and supportive love, as well as fear, pain, and the isolation of disease.

It seemed possible that those symbols in hospital which pointed to healing and personal integration could be an antidote to the negative effects of the disease itself in an understanding of life. We found that some people responded to the immediate symbols of love in their situations, whereas others could be helped best by exploring with them the symbols that had given them life in the past, or hopes for the future, so that these could be made effective in the present through counselling. This we called *symbolic therapy.*

Much of this is no more than common sense, and forms the basis of all counselling work. The ethos of the symbols of care is accepted as right for a hospital by almost everyone. Yet this does not in any way deny the validity of the symbols. Rather, it strengthens the idea by giving practical proof of its effectiveness. *Where symbolic theory does go beyond common sense is that it allows practical experience in hospital to become an element in the theological debate.*

Theology claims to be dealing with suffering and what faith means within it – and it must therefore see the *whole* situation, and not just the part of it that relates to the medical condition. It is complex, and contains both negative and positive sides.

79

The sense of companionship for a person who is often lonely, the care and concern of the medical and nursing staff, receiving cards and flowers from neighbours and friends, and the general fact of being cared for – all these may become positive symbols of hope, and they are just as real a part of hospital experience as the disease.

It should be possible to gain faith in a cancer hospital in the same way as it is gained anywhere else, by recognizing that certain truths are fundamental for life. *There are many ways in which the intensity of ward life, and the personal nature of the issues that are faced there, make a person more aware than normally of the real values and qualities of human life.* So much that is superficial in society is stripped away in the hospital.

We are not trying to give an assessment of the good and the bad within a hospital in order to get some balance or general conclusion. The failure of that line of approach has already been shown. This is existential. It is an assessment of those elements in the experience which speak to the individual person of his ultimate truth and value. And this will be understood differently by each person.

In its broadest sense, religion is a response to that which is seen as ultimately of value in terms of a distinctive pattern of life, and from this can come statements expressing what has been perceived. In the Christian religion, the focal point of the experience is the person of Christ. He points beyond himself to authentic human living for all, and expresses what it might mean in his own life.

The Christian faith therefore centres on symbols expressing the Christ experience, and these include his healing, his loving acceptance of all (and especially those who were socially out-cast), his willingness to risk personal suffering and his integrity in the face of great opposition. Springing out of them all is the symbol of *resurrection*, affirming triumph even in the face of apparent failure and execution, and the living reality and power of his life among those who follow him.

The Christian faith proclaims that the ultimate truth about human life is shown in humility, love and service, and comes to the fore *within* human fragility and suffering, and not in spite of it. We might therefore expect to see symbols of transcendent love in a situation of suffering, rather than in one of superficial success.

In the case history of a person suffering from cancer there will be many important things which never show up in the medical notes. These are the moments of human insight and truth, pointing to what life is really about. They are moments which proclaim that the most real thing is not suffering and disease, but *the person who is going through them*. Our concern for the cure of disease is at all points secondary to our concern for the person who is sick; and if it is *not*, then we are not practising medicine, but only playing with medical possibilities.

The symbols of value that appear within our situation may be resymbolized in terms of God. 'God' will be the name we give to the ultimate truths and depths of life that are revealed. It is an optional resymbolization, but a valuable one. It enables the depths of experience to be spoken about simply and directly.

Seen in this way, all who struggle for human beings and against disease affirm aspects of God, although they may find no reason to speak about 'God'. *To believe in a God of love is to declare that love is at the heart of true human living, and should be the ultimate motivation for all human activity*. The only atheist in these circumstances is one who is indifferent to the fact of human suffering, who sees health and disease as equally to be promoted. He is the person who has no scale of values or priorities in life, and cannot enter into the struggle against disease because he sees no point in working on behalf of people. For the true atheist nothing is worthwhile. Disease, pain and isolation do not matter, since health, compassionate removal of pain, and acceptance of an individual to overcome isolation have no value either.

This means that there can be very few atheists, and it is difficult to see how any can be found among those who work for the relief of suffering. Anyone who gives himself to the task of helping others, reveals his valuation of human life. It may never be resymbolized in terms of God, but it is no less real for that. What matters is that the transcendent dimension of ultimate human values continues to be perceived and to direct the course of those who work for the benefit of humanity.

However one describes the situation, there are within a hospital large numbers of patients, relatives and staff who care desperately about the value and quality of human life. They see situations every day in which these are revealed on the wards. They recognize that the value of human life is relevant to decisions about the use of medical technology, and through them faith grows and finds practical expression.

Any attempt to argue rationally from these things to an idea of God remains possible but rather futile. It is always inconclusive, whereas the reality of God is found day by day in the values expressed in the medical world.

The human situations in hospital, along with the past experiences that patients bring with them and the hopes that sustain them, are the raw material of human affirmation. If we recognize the symbolic nature of these things, and of the transcendent dimension in all life, then we can start to have a positive and creative approach to suffering. Through it much faith may be revealed and hope created, and each individual has much to discover and share with others. In this way, the times of fragility and disease, as well as those when all goes easily, provide the material upon which our understanding of what it means to be fully human is to be forged.

Appendix

Tillich on the Religious Symbol

Books by Tillich on the religious symbol are here listed in chronological order.

'Das religiöse Symbol', *Blätter fur Deutsche Philosophie*, 1928, translated as 'The Religious Symbol', *Journal of Liberal Religion* 2, 1940

The Religious Situation, New York 1932

'Symbol and Knowledge: a Response', *Journal of Liberal Religion*, Spring 1941

'Philosophy and Theology', *Theology* 44, 1942, pp. 132–43

'The Two Types of Philosophy of Religion', *Union Seminary Quarterly Review* 1, May 1946, pp. 3–13

'The Problem of Theological Method', *Journal of Religion*, January 1947

Systematic Theology 1, University of Chicago Press 1951 and Nisbet 1953

The Courage to Be, Nisbet 1952 and Collins Fontana 1962

'Autobiographical Reflections' and 'Reply to Interpretation and Criticism', in C. W. Kegley and R. W. Bretall, *The Theology of Paul Tillich*, Macmillan 1952

'Existential Analysis and Religious Symbols', in *Contemporary Problems in Religion*, ed. H. A. Basilius, New York 1954

'Theology and Symbolism', in *Religious Symbolism*, ed. F. E. Johnson, New York 1955

'Religious Symbols and Our Knowledge of God', *Christian Scholar* 128, 1955, pp. 189–97

'The Relation of Metaphysics to Theology', *Review of Metaphysics* 1956

Dynamics of Faith, Allen and Unwin 1957

Systematic Theology 2, University of Chicago Press and Nisbet 1957

'The Meaning and Justification of Religious Symbols' (1961), in S. Hook (ed.), *Religious Experience and Truth*, Oliver and Boyd 1962

Ultimate Concern, SCM Press 1965

Systematic Theology 3, University of Chicago Press 1963 and Nisbet 1964

Although spread over three decades, this material shows a remarkable consistency of thought. His last article was produced as a lecture for the New York Institute of Philosophy in 1960, but at the same time he distributed copies of 'The Religious Symbol', although it had been written in German in 1928. In the light of that, any slight alterations in language and terminology from one article to another are almost incidental.

Notes

Chapter 1

1. These details are taken from J. Walter, *Cancer and Radiotherapy*, Churchill Livingstone 1973.

2. Results as given in *Cancer and Radiotherapy*. All medical details have been checked as to their general validity, but apart from those quoted from a particular source they should not be regarded as having any medical authority.

Chapter 2

1. This situation is now modified for many of the younger patients at the Royal Marsden Hospital. Those under thirty are asked only to sign for a biopsy. If further surgery is then found to be necessary it is discussed with the patient afterwards. Those between thirty and forty are generally given a choice: either they can give permission for the surgeon to proceed if necessary, or they can have a biopsy only. This is intended to reduce the anxiety, especially in the large numbers of young patients with benign lumps, and to give more choice to the patient.

Chapter 3

1. This last figure is given in K. D. Bagshawe, *Medical Oncology*, Blackwell 1975. The earlier book, J. Walter, *Cancer and Radiotherapy*, 1973, gave it as only 40%. These and other figures are included in order to give a general impression of the situation. Except where their source is quoted, they claim no medical authority.

2. Much concern in this field has been promoted by the work of Dr Cecily Saunders at St Christopher's Hospice. Among the literature available is: John Hinton, *Dying*, Penguin Books 1967; Colin Murray Parkes, *Bereavement*, Penguin Books 1975; also articles by Richard Nicholson, R. G. Twycross and Michael Wilson, with a commentary

by C. M. Fletcher in *Journal of Medical Ethics*, Vol. 1, No. 1, April 1975. The above all carry valuable bibliographies.

Chapter 4

1. The theory of religious symbolism used in this section is based on that of Paul Tillich. A full list of his works on the subject is included here as an appendix.

2. This illustration is taken from Tillich's earliest article on symbolism, 'The Religious Symbol', *Journal of Liberal Religion* 2, 1940.

3. This was also Tillich's conclusion. In a footnote to p. 33 of 'The Religious Symbol' he wrote: 'The idea is that if God is all in all, there is no more need to speak of God in special symbols or even to use the word "God". Speaking of things would mean speaking of the depth in which things are rooted and of the heights to which they are elevated.' And as late as *Systematic Theology 3*, Nisbet 1963, he was still able to say: 'Every act of life should in itself point beyond itself and no realm of particular acts should be necessary' (p. 103).

Chapter 6

1. For a complete and detailed account of this problem see John Hick, *Evil and the God of Love*, Macmillan 1966 (references here are to the Fontana Books paperback edition 1968).

2. Ibid., p. 5.

3. James Martin, *Suffering Man, Loving God*, St Andrew Press 1969, p. 67.

4. C. S. Lewis, *A Grief Observed*, Faber and Faber 1961, p. 31.

Chapter 7

1. Antony Flew and Alasdair MacIntyre (eds), *New Essays in Philosophical Theology*, SCM Press 1955.

2. Ibid., pp. 96–9.

3. Ibid., pp. 99–103.